S0-DVF-208

Give Fat The Boot by Terry Joel

Copyright © 2008 Terry Joel. All rights reserved.

No part of this book or accompanying materials may be reproduced by any mechanical, photographic, or electronic process, or in the form of a phonographic recording, nor may it be stored in any retrieval system, transmitted, or otherwise copied or circulated for public or private use without prior written permission of Terry Joel.

This information and advice published or made available in this book is not intended to replace the services of a physician or health care professional.

Information in this book is provided for informational purposes only and is not a substitute for professional medical advice. You should not use the information contained herein to diagnose or treat a medical or health condition.

Please consult a physician in all matters relating to your health, and use discretion when practicing any of the exercises contained herein. The author and publisher make no representations or warranties with respect to any information offered or provided in this book regarding effectiveness, action, or application of the exercise and diet protocols contained herein. The author and publisher are not liable for any direct or indirect claim, loss or damage resulting from use of the information contained herein.

This book was printed in the United States of America.

To order additional copies of this book, please contact:
Golden Rule Press
Hackensack, NJ 07601
Phone: (201) 535 4475
Fax: (206) 984 4749

Table of Contents

Author's Thanks

If not for the loving support and encouragement of my beautiful wife, Diane, I would still be working at a job that was not leading to my growth as a fitness expert. Instead, since moving to California from South Florida, I have had the good fortune of working with several hundred people in the East San Francisco Bay area, and helping them to dramatically change their bodies and lives.

I owe thanks for my knowledge of physical fitness and weight management to the mentorship and guidance of some of the best experts in the world:

Dr. Anthony Abbott Ed.D, FACSM, CSCS*D

Without the solid foundation of fitness science and work ethic I learned from you, I would not have had the necessary foundation I needed to achieve depth in my understanding of all I have learned since attending your Fitness Institute International.

Juan Carlos Santana MED., NSCA-CSCS, Director of the Institute of Human Performance

You make the most complex concepts simple to understand and fun to learn. All of my programs and group camps strive to reflect your wisdom.

Phil Kaplan

My ability to utilize my education in my own business, where I have the opportunity to positively influence the lives of others, is thanks to the use of the outreach tools that you offer to any trainer who is committed to success.

<u>And My Clients</u>

You all continually inspire me to improve myself in order to remain worthy of your confidence and trust. Together, we will achieve miraculous results in our efforts for fitness.

Fitness and friendship,

Terry Joel (Coach Terry)
CPT-*National Strength and Conditioning Association*
Fitness Instructor, Certified-*American College of Sports Medicine*
CPTS-*Fitness Institute International*
Club Coach-*USA Weightlifting*

About Coach Terry

Terry Joel is the owner of Coach Terry's Health and Fitness in Concord, California and mentors the personal training staff development at Maverick's Sports Club in the same city. He not only personally trains clients in their pursuit of fitness and weight loss, but also is dedicated to raising the bar for all personal trainers in the East San Francisco Bay area. His exciting style combines the benefits of functional training with the fat loss and strength gains of traditional weights, securing thrilling results for those who experience his training approach.

Coach Terry has lectured around San Francisco at corporate offices and has been interviewed on ABC Channel 7's "View from the Bay." He holds certifications with the American College of Sports Medicine, National Strength and Conditioning Association, Fitness Institute International, and USA Weightlifting. At 59, Coach Terry is a living testament for what a healthy, active lifestyle can do to maintain a strong, sexy, and muscular body at any age.

Coach Terry's fitness lifestyle began in October 1973, when at the wise old age of 23 he woke up one morning and was guided to the conclusion that his unhealthy lifestyle was leading him in the wrong direction. A short run in the sand on North Miami Beach was followed by a visit to Lionel Playworld where he bought a small barbell and dumbbell set. It wasn't too long (one year) before the sickly 114 lb wise-guy was transformed into 125 lbs of lean muscle.

Today, Coach Terry is still growing physically and also spiritually. Fast forward through the body-building days of the 70's and 80's to today, and you will find he is sharing a great new education in exercise science and a passionate desire to help you understand how wonderful it is to be stronger than ever at 59 years old. Terry preaches the fitness truth to as many people as he can.

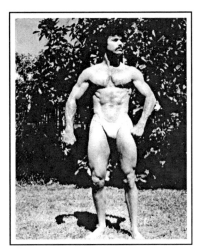

1980
31 years old
and healthy

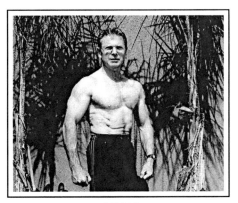

2005
56 years old
healthy and happy

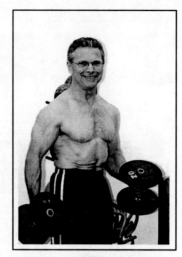

2008
59 years old and in
the best shape ever.

Introduction

Give Fat the Boot is a compilation of helpful fat-loss tips and my personal system that I use to program myself and my clients for success. Despite the saturation of the book market with hundreds of exercise and diet publications, there are precious few that address the highly effective technique of a program circuit that blends the best of functional training with the best of strength and conditioning.

In this book, you will learn how to create your own *Give Fat the Boot* circuit simply by picking your favorite exercises from one of four categories I have provided for you. In a short period of time, you can be your own fitness expert and enjoy the fabulous new body that you have designed and earned.

In my fitness journey of exercise and nutrition, I have tried many approaches from bodybuilding to long distance running to drinking some very unpleasant (but guaranteed effective) liquids. Having reached my goals and helped hundred of others do the same; I am a testament to the fact that your body can undergo a spectacular transformation at any age. Utilizing my experience and research, I am going to be your guide on one of the most remarkable transformations you have ever experienced.

My fitness program is a compilation of the best information, consolidated from the best conditioning and fat-loss experts in the world. I have been developing the philosophy of this program for about 15 years now and am confident in its effectiveness. Losing weight and getting fit goes way beyond dieting and exercising. It also requires a shift in your mind-set that is a prerequisite for success.

Unfortunately, most people do not recognize that about health, or they do, but the desire for instant gratification overrides any creative, solution-oriented thinking. The multi-billion dollar weight loss industry is all about "Lose weight – now!" with apparent apathy toward the long-term health of their customers.

I wrote this book, my first, wanting to provide a program of long-term health to you. My objective is not only for you to lose 10, 20, 50, or more pounds, double or even triple your energy levels, and have an unstoppable attitude. I would love to see you to happier in your body, get more done in less time, feel better physically and mentally, and substantially increase the quality of your life.

I know my goals are a lot to expect from a book, but you can have this kind of improvement. When you take care of yourself physically, you are better able to more quickly and easily service others and without resentment for using up your energy. In other words, *put yourself first*.

Taking care of yourself means properly fueling your body, challenging yourself physically, and growing and developing personally and professionally. We all want to achieve more, more easily, right?

We want more time, more money, more love, more fulfillment, more things, a better body, but we cannot gain all these things by only working out and watching what we eat. Diet and exercise are only a part of the whole you package.

Let us look at this in another way: if you are a very fit person and your diet is impeccable, but your life stinks, you are not likely to remain Mr. or Ms. Super-Fit for very long. Conversely, if you have a great life, but you let yourself go physically and your health is deteriorating, how can you possibly enjoy your wonderful life without any energy to do the things you want to do?

Give Fat the Boot is my approach to looking and feeling your best, covering all the bases in achieving complete health. You know you want to get there, which is why you are holding my book in your hands, so well done! You are off to a great start! The ball is now in your court.

If you are down in the dumps, have an unpleasant attitude, frequently start and stop diet and exercise plans, are getting discouraged, are out of shape, or your self-esteem is down the drain, your situation is more common than you probably think. In fact, these problems create a common, vicious cycle that leads to an inevitable downward spiral. Things can get better, because *Give Fat the Boot* is the solution that America has been waiting for.

With this book, you will get a clear tutorial on how to get the body of your dreams, be able to track your progress, and you will have accurate, helpful and modern information on your health in one source.

In this book, you have an exercise readiness page and health history form. If you have any risk factors or conditions that would make an exercise program dangerous for you, be sure to consult an experienced physician before beginning an exercise program.

You also have food guidelines that are based on practical nutritional knowledge and experience for healthy adults. I am not a registered dietitian and there are many experts who know more than I do about diets – do not hesitate to consult multiple resources in this area. To help you with this, I have included a list of the best nutritional experts, their books and websites.

Proceed to begin your journey to getting slimmer!

Fitness and friendship,
Coach Terry

Success Stories From People Like You

Back in New Jersey where I grew up, we learned real quickly that when people are selling something it is a lot easier to exaggerate than to show results. I have included a few letters from clients who, just like you, faced problems and challenges, but with patience and effort were able to achieve the body of their dreams.

Marlene's Adventure

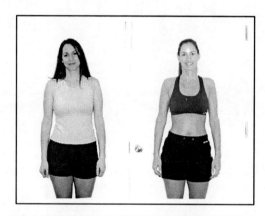

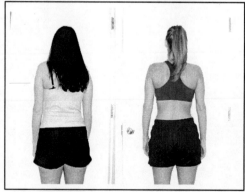

Coach Terry helped me to set my personal fitness goals at a reasonable and possible level. That didn't mean take this magic pill and in 24 hours all of the fat on your body will disappear, nor did it mean I could eat cookies all day without consequences. What this type of goal setting did do was help me to follow Coach Terry's plan of workouts one on one and join in on some group sessions. I ate a balanced meal of lean protein, starchy carbs, and fibrous carbs. And – watch out – I was on my way to a new me – a healthy, active, and slimmer me.

This simple of a plan sounds easy enough to do on your own, but Coach Terry throws in all of his years of expertise to help inspire and motivate you when it's not so easy to keep the cookies out of your mouth or when you don't feel like working out today or when the scale doesn't seem to move as fast as you would like it to because your fat is now turning into muscle!

Coach Terry always brings the workouts to my personal level, not too easy, but not so hard that I get hurt. He always makes sure I am exercising correctly with proper form for best results and to keep me safe. Coach Terry is the most educated trainer I know and he is always passing the latest information about nutrition and exercise to his classes, keeping us updated and informed. Coach Terry is very knowledgeable, and with knowledge comes power, and with power comes results that last a lifetime.

Thank you Coach, for teaching me how to be a stronger, healthier, slimmer me!

Marlene Mirabella
(a work in progress)

Rochelle's Fitness Goal Achieved

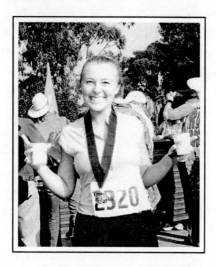

I was never on any particular diet or program before I started training with Terry – that is, unless bad eating habits count. I did try supplements such as HYDROXYCUT in hopes that a magic pill would melt away my body fat (yeah right); instead, they gave me the jitters and a racing heart rate.

Growing up, I would skip meals and eat small meals if I thought that I was plumping up too much. It wasn't until I was diagnosed with IBD that I started to take my health and habits more seriously.

A major challenge I have faced in my past regarding weight management and fitness was my family's history of bad eating habits and eating disorders. The women in my family have always been obsessed with the number on the scale, sometimes to the point of becoming anorexic or bulimic. I was always surrounded with comments on my weight regarding whether they thought I looked thin or not. I was never encouraged to play sports or to exercise to stay fit, so it was very challenging to learn to stay thin in a healthy manner. I was taught early in life to eat little or not at all.

My fitness level has improved dramatically since I have been training with Terry. Not only have I seen a difference in my physical appearance, but my techniques have improved and my endurance has increased. I have also advanced my knowledge of weight management and fitness.

My confidence and self esteem have grown, I feel healthier, my dreams have gotten bigger, and my goals have grown. I have fallen in love with my healthy life style and exercise. Terry has pushed me onto a whole different level that I thought I could never achieve. He has shown me that when I think I cannot go any farther, if I push a little harder, I will find that there are no real limits.

Training with Terry, I have learned to set high goals (realistically) and to strive for the best results for myself. I believe that I have improved my work performance and have moved forward in my career because of what I have learned from him. I plan everything out, whether it be for fun or for my career.

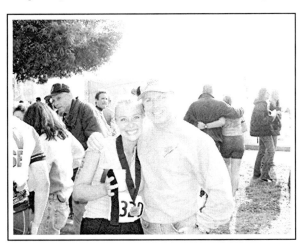

Terry is very encouraging and shows you how to get the best results by working with your techniques and posture. Terry always takes the time to make sure that his steps with you are perfect to help you achieve success from every angle. Terry does a wonderful job at encouraging me and motivating me.

Most importantly, he loves to see his clients improve and put their best efforts into his training methods. Terry is always on time and available for you. He loves his job and loves to see you improve in your everyday life, making success with Terry all but inevitable.

Thanks Terry!
Rochelle Cunningham

Alene's Incredible Four Month Extreme Make-over

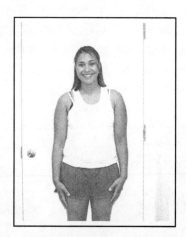

October 3, 2007
"Hey Coach, can you help me lose the weight that I haven't been able to lose since the birth of my baby girl?"

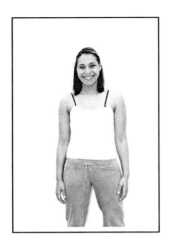

Week 11
December 19, 2007

"I'm fitting into jeans that I haven't been able to wear since my first trimester."

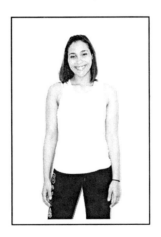

February 6, 2008

"Stay positive and motivated.
It's hard work but worth it.
Thanks Coach"

Oh, by the way, Alene is a busy single mom who still made it a priority to be successful at losing fat and reclaiming her beautiful figure.

The First Steps in Your Success Story

Your desire to possess the best body possible is the very first step in achieving just that. That you picked up this book shows your interest, but maybe you are uncertain of your potential at this early stage. I have included the testimonials in the preceding section to show you the potential that this program holds.

Marlene, Rochelle and Alene where unhappy with their bodies and came to me for help; now, they are athletes with strong, healthy bodies with which they are delighted. You can achieve the same results and be just as thrilled with your new body as they are with theirs.

Oh, by the way; Marlene is a busy mom with two beautiful daughters and a child-care business, and Alene is a single mom who had many challenges to overcome. If they can achieve phenomenal physical changes, so can you.

To make your fitness program work, you have to just do it. This chapter will help you to get motivated and reach your goals, because achieving the body of your dreams is simple. Simple is right, but notice that I did not say quick and easy like the infomercials claim. Positive physical change requires effort and education. Here is the success formula that works every time:

Supportive nutrition

+

Strength training

+

Moderate cardio

=

Nice Body

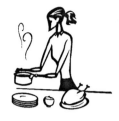

Supportive nutrition just means a diet that provides your body with the proper nutrients that you need to feed your muscles and burn fat. I will explain this more fully in a later chapter.

+

Strength training means challenging your muscles to grow bigger in order to burn more fat, just like a larger furnace burns more coal. You can use weights, bands, machines, or bodyweight to build your muscles. Following the teachings of this book, you can burn tremendous amounts of calories, build muscle, and learn how to move better.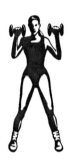

+

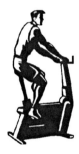

Moderate cardio (aerobic exercise) means just enough time in your heart rate zone to allow your body to get rid of more fat and not so much that you cannibalize lean muscle. I will also discuss how to make cardio more effective.

=

You looking in the mirror and seeing yourself slim and healthy in the best body that you ever thought you could have. This book contains all the information you need to make this happen for yourself.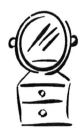

After the very first step of determining you want to make the effort and strive for physical perfection, but before jumping into what I have to teach you, you should take stock of your current situation. Take the time now to answer the following questions and record the answers both for your future reference when you are considering how much progress you have made in this program and to be certain that your health situation will not hinder you in your progress.

On the next few pages, I have included forms on which you can log useful information about yourself. The health history forms, which include a list of symptoms you need to be aware of before starting an exercise program, a list of risk factors for people who want to begin a fitness program, and a list of current health issues that will help you determine whether you are ready to begin an exercise program or if you should consult a physician first. When in doubt, consult first.

The personal and exercise information form and the measurements form give you space to record your goals and your starting points so you can compare your current fitness level to your measurements later on. By keeping these records, you will be able to measure the results of your fitness efforts, to keep in mind your fitness goals, and to be aware when you reach your goals.

One of the most important factors in your positive physical change will be your mindset – the absolute belief that you will stick to your empowering lifestyle and be successful. That is why I included some very important questions in the self-assessment readiness questionnaire that will help you to determine why change is important to you and what you are willing or not willing to do in order to stand on the gold platform of success. I urge you to take the time to fill these out fully and thoughtfully as they require you to consider parts of your thought processes and belief systems that may accelerate or slow your positive physical change.

Furthermore, if you do not already have a before picture, I highly suggest that you take one now. In a few weeks you will wish you had one.

Before photo	After photo

Health Questionnaire/Par-Q

Part I: Symptoms

Has your doctor ever said you have heart trouble, heart palpitation, coronary disease or high blood pressure?	
Do you frequently experience pain or discomfort in the chest or heart area?	
Do you suffer from shortness of breath at rest or upon mild exertion?	
Do you suffer from dizziness or fainting?	
Do you have any difficulty breathing?	
Do you suffer from swollen ankles due to circulation problems or a metabolic condition?	
Do you experience pain in your limbs when exercising or moving?	

If you answered "yes" to any of the above, please have your physician complete a medical clearance prior to exercise.

Part II: Risk Factors

Has a physician ever diagnosed you as having high blood pressure (greater than 170/90) or are you currently on blood pressure medication?	
(Optional) BP measurement: Right arm: _____ Left arm: _____	
Your cholesterol level is: _____ (less than 6 months ago). Is the value greater than 240 mg/dL?	
Do you smoke?	
Do you have diabetes?	
Has anyone in your immediate family suffered from coronary or atherosclerotic disease prior to age 55?	
Are you now or do you think you may be pregnant?	
If you answered "Yes" to two or more of the above, please have physician complete medical clearance before exercise.	

Part III: Medications/Limitations/Medical History

List any medications (and doses) you are currently taking:

_____
_____
_____

For what conditions?

_____
_____
_____

Do you have allergies? Y N   If so, what are they?

_____
_____
_____

Do you have any physical limitations that would limit your ability to exercise? Y N   If so what are they?

_____
_____
_____

List dates and reasons for/outcomes of any past surgeries, abnormal test results, hospitalizations, and/or treatments.

_____
_____
_____

Do you partake in regular physical activity? Y N   If so, how often?

_____
_____
_____

What types of activities?

_____
_____
_____

Part IV: Personal Information

Do you consider yourself overweight, underweight, or with no weight problem? _____
What do you consider a good weight for yourself? _____
What is the most you have ever weighed? _____
What changes would you like to make in your body composition? _____ _____ _____ _____ _____ _____
Exercise/Fitness Goals: _____ _____ _____ _____ _____ _____
Exercise History: _____ _____ _____ _____ _____ _____

Height:	_____	Weight:	_____
Resting Heart Rate:	_____	Maximal Heart Rate:	_____
Target Heart Rate:	_____	VO2 max (est.):	_____

Opinion of ideal weight:		_____
Age:	_____	
BP:	____ / ____	

Part V: Skin-Fold Measurements

(If you don't know how, or lack the calipers for these, then a good choice would be to see a professional trainer with a certification from NSCA or ACSM.)

Chest:		Triceps:	
Suprailiac:		Abdominal:	
Subscapular:		Midaxial:	
Mid-Thigh:		Bicep:	

All techniques for measuring body-fat inherently have a plus or minus percentage of standard deviation, whether you use hydrostatic weighing, calipers, or bio-impedance. (These are listed from the most accurate to the least.) The important thing is that they can reflect an accurate measure of *change* regarding loss of fat pounds. I don't recommend looking up the 4-, or 7-site conversion tables for percent fat until the second assessment when you have something to compare, thereby providing positive motivation rather than embarrassment.

Remember that the measurements that you take today are merely a starting point from which to measure your future success. Don't get all wrapped up in what the numbers are today. The only important numbers are those measured in the next 6 weeks and every 6 weeks after that.

Part VI: Progress Chart

	Test 1	Test 2	Test 3	Test 4	Test 5
Date					
Chest					
Shoulders					
Waist					
Abdominal					
Hips					
Thigh					
Calf					
Bicep					
Sum 7 sites					
Sum 4 sites					
Weight					
% Fat					
Lean mass					
Fat lbs.					
Fat loss					

Part VII: Self-Assessment Readiness Questionnaire

The following questions will help determine your level of readiness for change, your motivation towards reaching your goals, and identifying obstacles to your success.

Please answer each of the questions completely as these answers will help you to understand your major obstacles and find creative solutions.

1. Are you at some sort of health risk because of your current life style?

   _____
   _____
   _____
   _____

2. Are you seeking to make positive lifetime changes or achieving a short term temporary goal?

   _____
   _____
   _____
   _____

3. Are successes in small increments a motivator for you?

   _____
   _____
   _____
   _____

4. Are you willing to set realistic goals and prepared to deal with occasional setbacks?

_____

_____

_____

_____

5. Compared to previous attempts, how motivated are you at this time to change your lifestyle on a scale of 1-5?

_____

_____

_____

_____

6. Considering all outside factors at this time in your life (work, children, obligations etc.), what is your level of commitment to the time and effort involved in a body transformation program?

_____

_____

_____

_____

7. Have you already set aside the days and times that you can consistently be sure that you will be available to exercise and plan your nutrition?

_____

_____

_____

_____

8. Write down in detail all of the pain that you associate with being in your present condition.

_____

_____

_____

_____

9. Write why and how a lifestyle change will benefit you. Visualize clearly how this will look and feel.

_____

_____

_____

_____

The Easy Way, The Hard Way,
And Clearing Out The Misinformation

Nobody wants to work more than necessary to achieve fitness. In fact, at my age I want to know how little I need to do in order get maximum results, rather than how much. I need my programs to be effective, efficient and timely. But don't be fooled by the promises of infomercials and marketing campaigns that make fitness sound like something that does all the work for you.

Nothing works on its own. If a product or supplement promises to trim your tummy or give you the body of your dreams without including the synergy of strength training, moderate aerobics, and supportive nutrition, then you need to question the validity of those claims.

You can find examples of to-good-to-be-true inventions in almost every fitness magazine. Electric pulsing fat zappers, thigh trimmers, ab loungers, magic berry juices, and the list goes on. Anything you can do with a $2,000 "Blank-flex" machine can be done with a good quality resistance band, which is readily available for $24.

Magazines, infomercials, and self-proclaimed experts also give contradictory information about exercise in general. In order to get the most out of your exercise and out of your money, you need to know the truth about all these claims and put into practice what you know to be best for your fitness. I have included the truth about several exercise myths to keep you well-informed as well as corrections for common mistakes that beginning exercisers make. Be sure to study these myths and mistakes carefully to rectify any misconceptions you have about exercise. Knowing the truth and applying accurate information to your fitness program goes a long way in getting you as fit and healthy as possible in the best amount of time.

The Truth About Exercise

Exercise "tips" and programs come at us from all angles. Fitness has become a huge industry with all sorts of businesses and professions making big bucks off of our desire to be healthy. The wide range of information and misinformation we get from all sorts of people in our lives causes confusion and prevents maximization of our fitness efforts. By knowing the truth about exercise, you can utilize what you know and apply it to your new, healthy lifestyle.

Feminine Muscles Are Not Bulky

Sometimes women are concerned about the effects of strength-training on their looks. Most women do not want bulky muscles and, therefore, are concerned about exercising with weights. There is no need to worry about bulk, ladies. The women you see who are bodybuilders and are very bulky practice extreme measures to build those kinds of muscles. Many of them also take bulk enhancing drugs. Because women do not have much testosterone in their bodies, exercise – even intense exercise – has a slimming and healthy effect on their looks, not masculine consequences. By increasing your muscle mass and reducing fat you will be slim, sleek and sexy.

Extra Weight For Aerobic Exercise

Some joggers, walkers, and runners like to wear 1 or 2 pound weights on their arms and legs while they exercise. You would think this practice would help to build muscle and make the jogging, walking, or running more beneficial; but actually, adding small weights to your wrists and ankles is not worthwhile.

A couple pounds is not enough weight to achieve any of the benefits of strength training, while the extra pounds slow you down in your aerobic exercise. You aerobic workout needs to be intense for you to get the most benefit out of it, so you do not want to slow down, and, although you may feel like wearing weights is a good strength-training practice, this is not enough and cannot replace challenging weight work.

Trouble Spots

The typical person has a particular part of his or her body that is not liked by the owner. Whether your trouble spot is your thighs or your stomach, no matter how many squats or crunches you do, you cannot target the fat in that area for burning during exercise. Your fat is above your muscles, meaning that you cannot choose what fat you burn – only your genetics can do that.

You can, however, target muscles on your body. By targeting particular muscles, you can affect the tone and shape of that body part, helping it to look better and be stronger.

Weights: How Heavy

If you can lift a given weight more than 12 times *in perfect form*, then increase the weight. If the weights are lighter than this, they are not heavy enough to use for effective muscle growth (hypertrophy). Weights that are too light do not cause your muscles to strain sufficiently against the weight to build muscle. This means that, as you get stronger and the weights you are used to using become too light for you – when you can lift a weight more than 8 or 12 times in a row – you need to switch it out for a heavier weight to continue building your muscles.

On the other hand, if you can't perform at least eight repetitions with a given weight then it is too heavy and should be reduced. In advanced programs I will recommend changing the loads for every workout over the period of one week.

Losing Weight

Although most people expect to start losing weight as soon as they begin an exercise routine, the opposite is occasionally true. Some beginners gain a little weight before they start losing any. Exercising builds muscle and burns away fat. It is possible to add a *slight* increase since muscle is denser than fat while feeling slimmer and noticing that your clothes fit looser. With proper exercise intensity and food intake you should be able to expect one to two pounds of fat loss each week.

If you are doing plenty of exercise and still fail to lose fat then you are still eating too much, or sabotaging your fat loss with excess starchy carbs or sugar. It's that simple. Remember that there is a huge difference between weight loss and healthy, permanent fat loss.

Gain Through Pain

A lot of athletes appreciate a certain amount of soreness after a workout because muscle soreness is an immediate physical effect of their efforts, but much more pain than just a recognition of the progress you made can be a bad thing. There is no need to over-do your workout and risk burning out yourself on your fit lifestyle before even experiencing its real benefits. Don't work out so hard that you get so sore you don't want to exercise again or go back the next day for cardio intervals. This will actually work against your best intentions to be consistent.

Furthermore, if you go into a workout with any substantial amount of pain, you risk favoring a particular muscle group or protecting another, which can lead to poor form and possible injury. Be sure to always challenge yourself, but the object is to push your limits, not dangerously go past them. You do not need to experience large amounts of pain to experience the benefits of exercise.

Moderate-intensity exercise is just as beneficial to your health (although not necessarily to your physique) as high-intensity exercise, so don't make yourself not enjoy working out. Fitness is not an overnight achievement, but a significant, rewarding process that takes time and patience.

Common Mistakes

There is a great deal of misinformation floating around compliments of TV Infomercials and the multi billion-dollar diet industry. They would have you believe that fitness and weight management is quick and easy or that little effort is involved. These are a few common errors that sabotage results. You need to be aware of these mistakes to avoiding falling victim to false "tips."

Not Training with Enough Weight to Make a Difference

Within proper progression, you must challenge the muscles in a way that they are not used to in order to grow lean muscle and burn fat. If you have been using the same amount of weight on most exercises for a long time, then you are due for an increase in intensity. As I mentioned above, if you can lift a weight more than 8 or 12 times, you need to increase its weight in order to build strength and lean fat burning muscle.

Thinking that Regular Daily Activities Count as Exercise

Remember that your body adjusts to the actions you perform every day. This also goes for the same type of aerobic class that you may have been doing for a long time. If your job is labor-intensive or if you regularly perform the same exercise routine, while these habits are not harming you, they are not giving you the full benefit of exercise, either. Your body has figured out how to do what used to require a lot of calories, more efficiently. You need variety in your workout to avoid your body's adaptation to the strain, which prevents the best muscle strengthening and calorie burning.

Eating Too Little or Skipping Breakfast

A 130 pound woman will burn close to 1300 calories per day just by waking up and sitting on the couch. When you add exercise or daily work, then your daily basic calorie needs go up. When you eat less than your body needs to survive, you will slow down your metabolism and gain more fat. Supportive nutrition combined with exercise will speed up your metabolism and make you slimmer. Skipping meals – especially breakfast – will not help you to achieve your fitness goals, but will actually sabotage your efforts.

Hours of Working Out or Cardio Every Day

Just like nutritious food, the right thing is good, but too much food makes us fat. The right amount of exercise is good, but over training will ultimately break down muscle tissue, reduce your immune function, and lead to set-backs. Don't overdo your exercising efforts – be patient and consistent, not reckless or anxious. The great fat loss expert Alwin Cosgrove states it this way, "More isn't better; Better is Better."

Slow Cardio Exercise

If you read the panels on most aerobic machines, you may be led to believe that if you spend a lot of time moving slowly, then fat will magically disappear from your body. This is a myth based on distorted information. People burn a greater percentage of fat calories doing lower intensities of exercise, but this does not mean that you will burn more fat by doing slow exercises. There is a big difference between percentages and actual amounts. In fact, the largest percentage of fat calories burned is at rest.

Your body is always burning the various fuels in your body, usually a mixture of fats and carbohydrates. When you are resting, you probably burn about 70 percent fat and 30 percent carbs. When you are active, however, the percentage changes, and your body burns a larger percentage of carbs. The more physically intense your activity, the lower the percentage of fat in the mix of burning fuels, until the percentage reaches approximately 99 percent carbohydrates and 1 percent fat. Although 1 percent seems much lower than 70 percent, you will burn much more fat with an intense exercise than with a low-intensity exercise.

If you were offered 70 percent of the savings of the next teenager you met or 1 percent of the wealth of the United States, which would you choose? Obviously, the 1 percent, although percentage-wise is much lower, quantity-wise is much, much higher. Therefore, even though the percentage of burned fat calories during rest or slow exercise is high, the actual amount of fat burned is minimal and will not make you much slimmer. You need to crank up the intensity if you want to see your six-pack anytime soon.

Cardiovascular Exercise

I also have some interesting news for you regarding cardiovascular activities: they do not lead to much fat loss over time. Also, since the body quickly adapts to any activity done repeatedly, you can slow down your metabolism by doing too much cardiovascular activity. If they do not burn a lot of fat and can possibly slow down your metabolism, why should you do them?

Cardiovascular exercise, often called cardio, is moderate aerobic exercise that strengthens your for heart, lung, and circulatory health. The benefits of increased circulation, efficiency of the heart as a pump, and increased mitochondrial density (fat burning factories in your cells) are significant and proven. Your lungs can also enjoy the increased ability to utilize oxygen, which is good for you all the way around. Therefore, cardio exercise is a must-do for your health, even though cardio can be challenging for a beginner.

The Most Important Thing to Know About Cardio

You will be much more likely to achieve your goals by performing intense interval training on your cardio of choice in the form of one minute very hard, followed by two minutes of mild to moderate intensity. For example, if you are on a treadmill, a speed and incline that produces a very uncomfortable feeling of breathlessness after one minute would be followed by a minute of getting your breath back at a slower, lower setting. Then, a minute of moderate before ramping the level back up again. It doesn't matter which type of cardio based activity you use, so go ahead and use the elliptical, Airdyne bike or run up hills for intervals.

Repeating this sequence six to ten times will transform your mindless cardio sessions into a challenging workout that will jack up your metabolism and induce your body to burn more fat for the next 14-18 hours. This is the result of excess post workout oxygen consumption (EPOC). This method will achieve a *nine times* faster weight loss than traditional cardio. You will read more about this in the chapter on boosting your metabolism.

How to Get the Most Out of Your Program

The benefits of having a leaner body – a body with more quality muscle – are explained throughout this book and everywhere in the media, but you need to know how to build this kind of muscle to gain those benefits. You need to know the difference between training for a long time as opposed to training efficiently for maximum fat loss.

How many sets and reps should you do with how much weight and how long you should wait before you do your next set are all pieces of information you need to know to be able to utilize the exercises you will learn in this program.

I have included a list of frequently asked questions and their answers for you to better know how to utilize what you learn from this book for the benefit of your body.

1. How long do I wait before my next set?

If you are using my 3 or 4 exercise circuits, by the time you have completed your other three exercises, your body will be more than ready to resume your main exercise of the circuit. Your transition time to get from one exercise to the next should be within 30 seconds.

2. Which exercises should I perform first?

For safety, always do the skilled and explosive exercises like snatch, power cleans, and clean and jerk in the beginning of a session while you are fresh and loaded with energy. Fatigue leads to dangerous imperfection of proper technique, which often leads to injury and weakness. Plyometric types of activities like box jumps can also be added to this list. Those who are not doing those types of lifts can begin with compound lifts like squats, bench-press, lat pulls, and dead-lifts to work major muscle groups at the beginning of the exercise session.

3. What is resistance training?

Resistance training is a common type of strength training for developing the strength and size of skeletal muscles. Weight training uses the force of gravity in the form of weighted bars, dumbbells, or weight stacks to oppose the force generated by muscle through concentric or eccentric contraction. Weight training uses a variety of specialized equipment to target specific muscle groups and types of movement.

4. What is Functional Training?

Functional training is simply training the body as a unit, rather than separating parts on different days. The training environment is in all planes of motion and 360 degrees around, creating a more harmonious, injury resistant, muscular appearance with the added benefit of enhanced movement skills and sports performance.

5. What is good form?

Each exercise has a specific form, or topography of movement designed to maximize safety and muscle strength gains. Going to technical failure on a set of exercise is always safer than struggling to get more reps than your body is capable of performing perfectly. Technical failure simply means that you can't produce another repetition in absolutely perfect form.

6. What is a rep?

Rep is short for repetition. A rep is a single cycle of lifting and lowering a certain weight in a controlled manner, moving through the form of the exercise.

7. What is a set?

A set is the number of repetitions completed in good form. Depending on the individual goal, a set can be 4-6, 8-12, or 15-25 or more repetitions.

8. What is maximum (RM)?

RM is an abbreviation of a maximal effort for a repetition of an exercise. A one rep-max is the most weight that a person can lift for a given exercise *in good form.* I rarely test for 1RMs because they carry undue risk, and for most people they are irrelevant. A much safer version is a three or four rep-max which can easily be mathematically converted to a 1RM equivalent.

9. What is tempo?

Tempo is the speed with which an exercise is performed. For example, lowering the bar to a count of 4 seconds in a bench-press and raising it to a count of 2 (4/2); or lowering in a 3 count, pausing 1 second and raising in 1 second (3/1/1). The tempo of a movement has implications for the weight that can be moved and the effects on the muscles. Tempo is important because it helps you gain muscle by increasing time under tension for the exercise performed.

Emotional/Chemical Benefits of Exercise

Within your body, when you experience stress, there is a chemical reaction called the fight or flight reflex. Long ago, when humans faced stress the situation was usually a physical threat to their well-being. In order to prepare you for this physical confrontation, your body produces the hormone cortisol. If cortisol is not burned off in a physical fight, your body stores it. Since stressful situations typically do not culminate in physical fighting these days, your body rarely burns off the cortisol. Instead, your system stores the cortisol, leaving it to potentially damage your body.

The physical activity of exercise simulates the action of fighting, giving your body the opportunity to burn off these unhealthy chemicals without the unhealthy fight. Aerobic exercise removes cortisol from your body, expelling the harmful hormone as well as your negative emotions. In general, exercise relaxes both your mind and your body, providing you with a perfect method to perform the vital physical activity for which your body and its systems are built.

There are other chemical reactions within your body that are helpful instead of harmful to your well-being. Exercise stimulates many of these. Physical activity causes your body to increase its production of serotonin neurotransmitters, norepinephrine hormone neurotransmitters, and dopamine hormone neurotransmitters. You may recognize dopamine from drug commercials – this hormone regulates your feelings of pain, well-being, pleasure, motivation, sleep, attention, learning, and mood. Serotonin helps you to control your mood, sleep, anger, aggression, sexuality, and appetite. And norepinephrine increases your heart rate. As you can see, these chemical reactions to exercise are immeasurably beneficial to you. In fact, the benefits of exercise are so great for your feeling of well-being that physical activity is often used as an effective treatment for depression.

Furthermore, because exercise helps your body to work as efficiently as possible, exercise significantly boosts your energy level. Exercise even increases your self-confidence. Exercise allows you to separate yourself from your day and your environment to focus on yourself and your well-being. During exercise, your mind is stilled and your body focuses you on repetitive, steady actions, allowing you to sort of re-boot and almost meditate during your workout. There is actually no difference between a good meditation session and a perfect set of squats.

Metabolic Stimulation:
Your Ticket to Fat Loss and a Body Your Friends Will Envy

The reason that most people are fooled into believing in nutty diets or infomercial products is because they really haven't been informed what really happens to fat in the body.

The Only Way Fat Leaves Your Body

(Skip over this part if you never want to know how to make more informed choices regarding your exercise and food choices.)

Mobilization:

Let's take a good look at your fat cells and what gets them excited. Well, there are two things really. One is the presence of a meal, and the second is a response to exercise. In order for a fat cell to be reduced, the stored triglycerides must first be broken up into free fatty acids (FFA's) and transported with a protein escort to a muscle cell to be burned as energy. This job is designated to the enzyme, Hormone Sensitive Lipase (HSL), which enters the fat cell and separates the FFA's.

Two main hormones can affect HSL and subsequent fat mobilization, insulin and the catecholamines. Insulin is the main inactivator of HSL and it takes only small amounts to mess up your progress. Catecholamines are energy hormones that travel through the bloodstream and under the right circumstances, stimulate HSL. Catecholamines are released as a response to exercise.

The take home message is that insulin will always block fat cell metabolism regardless of catecholamine

58

levels and will suppress HSL. Insulin spikes result from sugar and excess starchy carbohydrate intake.

Transport:

So once the FFA's are in the bloodstream, they need to be escorted to a muscle cell to be burned with oxygen. Owning an efficient circulatory system is one of the benefits of "Cardio for Health." We also get them from any challenge to the muscles requiring us to breathe harder and boost the heart rate.

Oxidation:

The final stage of fat's journey is to the mitochondria of muscle cell. Mitochondria are simply the fat burning factories in every cell. We actually can increase the fat burning factories in our cells by 15-35% as a result of doing cardio vascular exercise.

Mitochondria are also capable of growing by up to 15% which can give you another added boost in the fat fight. Taking a five minute rest after a hard work-out or interval session will allow a huge amount of FFA's to be dumped into the bloodstream. Follow the break with 20-40 minutes of steady state cardio for health and the muscles will use them for fuel. All it takes to block your knockout punch to fat is sugar.

This might not be like the most exciting thing that you have ever read, but understanding it is crucial to fat loss success.

More Metabolism Building Strategies

There are various ways to boost your metabolism. I have mentioned many of them throughout this book; here are some more for you to utilize in burning away your excess fat.

Cardio Based Intervals

This is one of the most effective fat loss methods available today. After a three to five minute warm-up at a slow pace; simply perform one very hard minute of your cardio of choice followed by two easy minutes. The hard minute should leave you feeling uncomfortably out of breath but still able to recover regular breathing and a lowered heart rate within a minute.

Repeat from 5-10 times, then rest 5 minutes and finish with 20-30 minutes of steady state cardio to burn off the now circulating free fatty acids.

You can use any favorite cardio based activity to create an intense interval workout. For example, a hard minute of running fast on a treadmill followed by the two easier minutes.

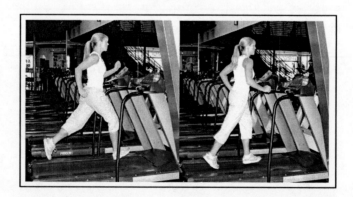

You might also use an Airdyne bike, which is one of my favorites.

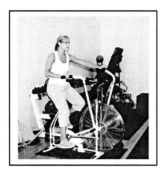

Or run line drills on a basketball court or field. My other favorite is simply to run up a hill for a minute and walk down for two minutes.

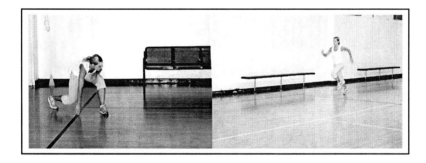

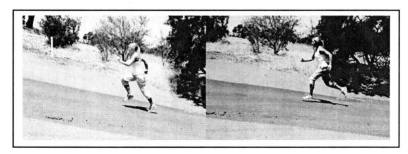

Strength Training Intervals

Intervals do not necessarily need to be cardio-based exercises for them to be effective. In fact, whenever you place at least four exercises in a circuit, you get a similar effect because your heart rate will soar when your muscles perform the exercises, then will lower between them.

For example, when you do a set of squats followed by standing press, lat pull-downs, and high to low chops, this circuit can be considered an intense interval. Follow the last exercise with about 30-60 seconds of rest, and then repeat for 3-5 sets. This is how I train myself and my clients most of the time. Sometimes I even stick a cardio exercise in between to elevate my heart rate.

Below is a circuit showing a level change (squat), push (military press), pull (Lat pull-down), and rotation (high to low chops). I provide more examples of this in the programming section of putting it all together.

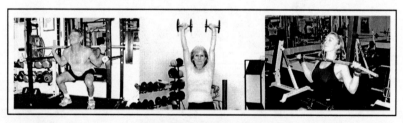

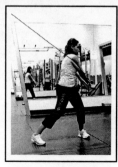

Intensive Exercise Classes

Many people are going outdoors and enjoying roughing it up outside in boot-camp style exercise classes, such as my "Give Fat the Boot" class. You can create your own class and have a blast doing it just by taking advantage of your mastery of the 4 pillars of human motion and making a 10-14 station circuit of exercises that have 2 or 3 of each type. Spend 40-50 seconds on each exercise, allowing for a 15 second transition. Get your breath back in between stations. You will be pleasantly tired in less than an hour if you repeat the circuit three times.

The other exciting advantage is that you have worked all of your body parts thoroughly while addressing strength, movement skills, agility, flexibility, and the ability to burn fat for a long time after. In my *Give Fat the Boot* class, this idea has been refined to the point that the classes are always fresh since there are so many examples of each of the 4 pillars combinations to choose from. I have included a complete example of a 12 exercise circuit in the *"Circuit Training: Putting the Exercises Together"* section on page 112.

Metabolic Challenges
Use these exercises in your own circuits to boost your metabolism:

Super Leg Circuit
This metabolic challenge will provide the ultimate in leg development. Three sets, twice per week results in fantastic legs for the rest of your life. If you are a beginner you will need to reduce the repetitions of the sequence to 10/10/10/5 adding two additional

repetitions per week until you are up to the 24/24/24/12.

1. 24 Speed Squats: Use excellent squat form and go as low as you can to make these effective

2. 24 Lunges: Maintain the hands behind the neck position to get a beneficial anterior torso and hip flexor stretch as you perform these.

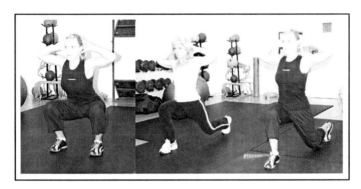

3. 24 Alternating Split Plyo Squats: Explode off the front leg alternating in mid air to land with the opposite leg in the front. This can also be performed on a box or a high step.

4. 12 Squat Jumps: These will feel like a huge burn in your thighs so keep going and finish strong. From a perfect squat, jump as high as you can and land back into the perfect squat position.

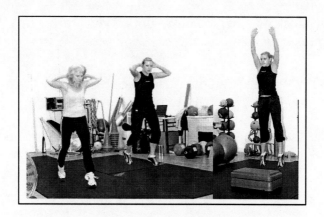

Super Chest/Arm Circuit

I often use this as the cornerstone of my chest, shoulder and triceps development. I always get people coming up to me and asking what I have been taking to get so big and defined. They are usually amazed when I just tell them that all it takes is a medicine ball and a lot of guts and time to progress. Start with 3/3/3/3 and progress by one extra rep per week until you own the whole sequence for three sets.

1. 5)ne-Arm Lockout Push-ups: Keep your knees, hips, abs, and head in line. Push hard with the hand that is on the ball to extend the arm completely. The free hand should come off the floor to a point level with the one on the ball. Repeat with the opposite arm.

2. 5 Over the ball Push-ups: Staying in proper alignment as before, follow your last lock-out with 5 on each side over the ball push-ups.

3. 15 Two Hands on Ball Push-ups: Be sure to continue staying in alignment with your butt tucked in and your core stiff. Lowering your elbows toward your belt until you touch the ball with your sternum

66

instead of your chest will maximize triceps and shoulder involvement. Avoid letting your arms flare out to the side.

4. 5 Plyo Push-ups: Now that your arms are very tired we will ask them to do more. Follow your last push-up by jumping off the ball and quickly jumping right back on. Controlling the ball so that it doesn't roll away from you is part of the exercise.

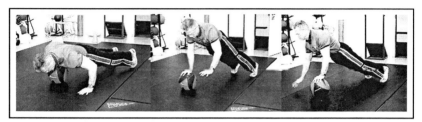

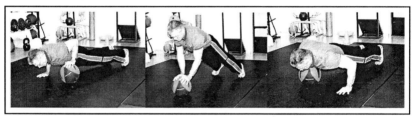

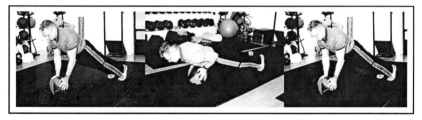

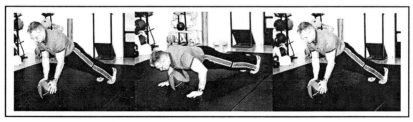

Super Back

Use a J.C. Band of medium to heavy thickness for this series of exercises that will build and strengthen your back and biceps muscles.

1. Two-hand Parallel Stance Rows: Stand far enough from the anchor to create a challenging resistance then perform 20 rows with both arms simultaneously. Be sure to pull back as far as you can and squeeze your shoulder blades together in the back.

2. Bent over Alternating Rows: Bend over and pull the bands alternately with one arm, then the other as shown.

3. Poling: Grasp the handles slightly above your chest in front with your arms fully extended. Then, forcefully press your arms down and back while flexing the trunk. This works the lats, long head of the triceps, and abs.

4. Medicine Ball Slams: Quickly drop the bands, and with a heavy medicine ball or dead ball, bring the ball high over your head and slam it down on the floor as hard as you can. Be sure that if it is a ball that will bounce, aim it away from your (or anyone else's) body.

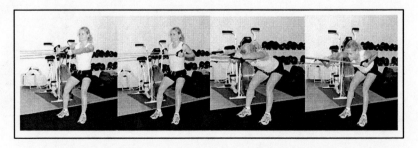

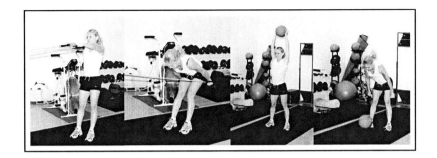

Super Abs

This series will carve your six-pack very quickly, provided you eat right and give it all you've got.

1. 15 Medicine Ball Crunches: From a supine position hold the medicine ball above your head and crunch.

2. 15 Medicine Ball Leg Lift: Place the ball between your feet and lift the ball up.

3. Medicine Ball Exchange: Combine the two previous exercises by placing the ball near your feet then leg then extend your body back to the straight position before you V-up to retrieve the ball with your hands. Repeat 15 times.

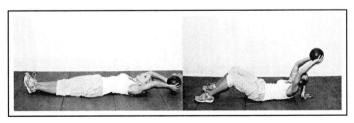

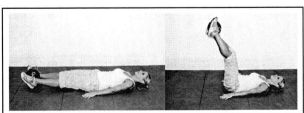

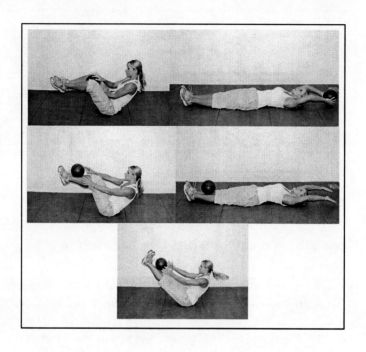

Stay Energized

Having enough energy to get through the day is something with which we all struggle. Each day is another struggle to accomplish everything on our to-do lists; if we do not have enough energy just to last the day, we tend to lose the struggle. There are many small changes you can make in your life that will boost your energy levels and avoid that afternoon yearning for a nap. By following these suggestions, you can raise your energy levels higher than you thought you could with any amount of caffeine.

Nutrition

First and foremost, never skip breakfast. If you eat fruit with other foods for breakfast, you are being especially helpful for your energy levels. Following this up by eating plenty of vegetables during lunch and dinner can keep the benefits going.

Regardless of how sincerely you love your morning coffee fix, however, energy does not come in a can or cup. Coffee and caffeine drinks just stimulate your central nervous system and mask fatigue.

The only effective way to fuel the body for energy is to ingest good carbohydrates, which provide your body with the energy it needs. Oatmeal (not instant oatmeal) with some nuts, blueberries, and non-fat yogurt will give you tons more energy for the day than two whole cups of coffee. A quarter cup of trail mix in a baggie can get you through a busy morning much better than anything that you can get out of the office candy machine.

In fact, eating sugar may give you a buzz at first, but it will lower your energy levels quickly after, making you worse off than you were before you snacked. Sugar ranks incredibly high on the glycemic index, meaning that your body burns through it very quickly, leaving you not only without an energy stimulant, but with an energy crash from your brief sugar high.

Eating white flour products has the same negative effect as eating sugar. Muffins, bread, pasta, and all your favorite cookies do horrible things to your blood sugar level and lead to a crash in your energy levels. As discussed in the nutrition chapter of this book, protein is an excellent provider of long-lasting high energy levels, especially if eaten in smaller amounts throughout the day. Foods high in fiber help you to maintain high energy levels and also help to prevent constipation, which is detrimental to your energy level.

As mentioned throughout this book, eating 5 - 6 meals a day is the most effective way to give your body the nutrients you need. By eating small meals throughout the day, you avoid the tiredness that follows a large meal and you regularly provide your body with energy sources.

When you eat a large meal, your body has to work to digest it – digestion is not as simple as just getting the food into your body. Because of this process, your energy levels drop after a large meal as your energy is being expended on digestion. Eating small meals, however, avoids any difficulties in digesting, avoiding a lull in your energy after a meal. Furthermore, eating healthy meals throughout the day constantly provides your body with a source of nutrients and energy that you can steadily use throughout the day without peaks and dips in your energy level.

Hydration

In addition to the food and food amounts that you give your body, being aware of the water you give your body can do wonders for your energy levels. There are countless reasons to stay hydrated, and one of them is to maintain energy. If you do not give your body enough water, your blood does not have enough water in it and circulation is not as effective as it should be. This causes the brain to not get all the nutrients and oxygen it needs to work efficiently, so you may start yawning, craving sugar, and become very tired as the brain tries to reach the oxygen levels it needs. Don't wait until you feel thirsty – drink at least 5-8 glasses of water throughout the day.

Even mild dehydration can drain away your energy and cause fatigue. Water is a vital element of every system in your body. In fact, 60 percent of your weight is from water, one of the most important components of your body.

Signs of dehydration include dark urine, dry mouth, dizziness, and skin tenting. (If you pull up the skin on your hand and it stays "tented" this indicates dehydration.)

Activity

Exercise, the cure for many of your ailments, also improves your stamina. Aerobic exercise does amazing things for your brain function and physical stamina, stimulating your body's production of feel-good hormones as well as better circulation, leading to an enhanced energy level. Exercising regularly will keep your energy levels higher than they are now. For a quick fix when you are feeling tired, just moving around can do a lot for your energy level.

There is something to be said about relaxation, too. For a quick fix, you can take a few minutes to just relax and occupy your mind with something purposeless. Being relaxed and focused can help you to overcome feelings of tiredness.

Deep breathing rejuvenates your system and brings energy-providing oxygen to your body. When you need to refresh your energy, sit or stand up straight and breathe very deeply – into your stomach, not your chest. Your cells need oxygen to function properly, so giving them the boost of oxygen they are yearning for results in the boost in energy that you want.

Stretching is a great physical exercise that can boost your energy without too much inconvenience. Stretching gets your blood flowing better, moves the oxygen in your body, and releases the tension and soreness you have built up throughout the day, leaving you feeling energized.

Absorbing sunlight is a great source of energy. Not getting enough sun can lead to fatigue, depression, and muscle weakness as well as some very serious illnesses, including osteoporosis and low vitamin D sufficiency. There are certain vitamins that your skin makes for which sunlight is a vital ingredient. Be sure to protect yourself from too much sun, but never neglect the sun as an important energizing and nourishing source.

Obviously, sufficient sleep is vital to your energy levels. Everyone needs a little different amount of sleep, but in general, you need 7 to 8 hours of sleep a night. Avoid caffeine for about 10 hours before you go to bed to help you to sleep sounder and more quickly. Be sure that your bedroom is dark because light interferes with your sleep, preventing your sleep from being as restful as it could be and as beneficial as you need your night's rest to be.

Last but not least, planning something for you to look forward to is a great way to up your energy. Planning a trip or starting a fun project can give you renewed vigor and excitement.

If you follow any or all of these tips, you will see marked improvement in your energy levels and will no longer by daunted by a long workday or exhausting schedule.

Your Training

Whether you have been exercising for a long time or are just beginning a program for strength training and weight management, you need to understand how the body adapts to exercise over periods of time. Years ago, we used to be taught that as you got stronger you needed to add more and more weight to your exercises in a linear fashion in order to achieve goals. We were also taught that we needed to push ourselves to the limit on every set of every workout (No Pain–No Gain Theory). The results of this type of strategy have been well-documented numbers of strains, rotator cuff injuries, joint impingements, and over-training syndrome.

Thanks to the Russian and Bulgarian Olympic champions, we now have accurate scientific methods to design programs that promote regular progress over time and avoid injury and staleness. These programs are based on the concept of *periodization*, or *cycling*, your training. There are volumes of ways to adjust your plans to help you to achieve specific results. I am going to focus on one plan that has worked for my clients and me for years. You can apply this plan as a beginner or as an elite athlete.

The training year consists of three cycles, which include several phases. In a simplified plan, I use 3 goal-oriented phases in a block.

- Condition/Tone = Adaptation 2 Weeks: this period prepares the body for the harder work to follow in the next cycle. In this cycle, I usually use a weight that allows the major exercises be lifted for 15-25 repetitions.

- Hypertrophy/Build = Larger Fat Burning Muscles 4-8 weeks: in this cycle, use more weight for major muscle groups in the range of 8-12 repetitions.

- Strength/Strength = Neural and Muscular Ability 2-4 Weeks: in this cycle, lift a rep range of 4-6 avoiding the overloading and risk of 1-rep maxes.

Sometimes in the art of programming yourself or with the guidance of a performance expert you will occasionally blend components of two or more phases to produce a desired performance or fat loss result.

After successfully completing a 13-week period, you are ready to begin again, but now you have changed to a new body that is stronger and more muscular, so your 15-25 reps will begin with slightly higher resistance than last time. You will also find the later parts of the other phases requiring more weight in order to challenge you to greater rewards.

Undulating Periodization

Another very effective way to manipulate training is simply train for hypertrophy (8-12) on Monday, strength (4-6) on Wednesday and conditioning on Friday (15-20). This method has been shown to be a great tool in our fat loss/muscle gain arsenal.

Cardiovascular Training

For your cardio (30 minutes after strength training and 1 hour on alternate days), be sure to track your time. Borg Rating of Perceived Exertion Scale (RPE) is *your* feeling on a scale of 20 regarding how hard the session was. For exercise purposes, the scale only needs to begin at 6 and end with 20.

As a reference, remember that 9 is comparable to a slow walk for a healthy person and 20 is so strenuous that most people never experience that intense of exercise. The scale is as follows:

Level Number	Amount of Exertion
6	no exertion at all
7	extremely light
8	
9	very light
10	
11	light
12	
13	somewhat hard
14	
15	hard (heavy)
16	
17	very hard
18	
19	extremely hard
20	maximum exertion

Your present condition will determine how hard an exercise seems and will change as you make positive changes in your body.

This subjective training guide is often a better method than objective training. The subjective style takes into account your physical and emotional state in determining your individual workout intensity rather than relying on an objective (arbitrary, really) percentage of age-predicted maximum heart rate.

Maximize Fat Loss Using Cardio Intervals

After a brief warm up at a light intensity, switch to a hard to very hard exercise for 1 minute, followed by 2 minutes of light to somewhat hard. Ten sets of this sequence will take about 30 minutes. Follow this with 5 minutes rest, then 20 minutes of regular, somewhat hard exercise. Finish with a 5 minute cool down to reset your heart rate to under 110 beats per minute. This interval training will transform boring cardio time to a fun workout and increase your body's ability to lose fat *all day long. I will mention this in more detail later.*

Sample Strength Training Log

Date: September 23, 2006

Exercise	Set 1	Set 2	Set 3	Set 4	Set 5
Squats	95/12	135/10	185/8	185/8	
SB – triple treats	BW/12 ea.	BW/12 ea.	BW/12 ea.	/	/
SB – crunches	/15	/15	/15	/	/
	/	/	/	/	/
bench press	95/12	115/12	125/8	135/8	/
lat pulls	90/12	110/10	130/8	130/8	/
low to high chops	20/10 ea.	20/10 ea.	20/10 ea.	/	/
	/	/	/	/	/
t-stabilizations	BW/10 ea.	BW/10 ea.	BW/10 ea.	/	/
SL/DB dead-lift	20/10 ea.	20/10 ea.	20/10 ea.	/	/
ABC extensions	Band/ 30 sec.	Band/ 30 sec.	Band/ 30 sec.	/	/
Cardiovascular exercise:	Cross-trainer				
Time:	20 minutes				
Heart rate:	146				
Rate of perceived exertion:	7				

What I did well: _I increased my weight on the bench press_
by 10 pounds and had better balance on the single dead lift
_____

What I would like to improve: _5 intervals of 1 minute hard_
and 2 minutes regular intensity would have been more
effective for fat loss _____

I have included a blank exercise log on the following
page for your own use. Feel free to make copies of the
log so that you can use this format continually.

Strength Training Log

Date: _____

Exercise	Set 1	Set 2	Set 3	Set 4	Set 5
	/	/	/	/	/
	/	/	/	/	/
	/	/	/	/	/
	/	/	/	/	/
	/	/	/	/	/
	/	/	/	/	/
	/	/	/	/	/
	/	/	/	/	/
	/	/	/	/	/
	/	/	/	/	/
	/	/	/	/	/
	/	/	/	/	/
	/	/	/	/	/
	/	/	/	/	/
	/	/	/	/	/
	/	/	/	/	/

Cardiovascular exercise:	Time: _____	RPE: _____		

What I did well:

What I would like to improve:

The Mechanics of Exercise:
How Movements Build Muscles

Total body conditioning has come a long way since 12 years ago, when we first heard the terms functional training and core exercise. In the 1970s and 1980s, gyms were packed with bodybuilding machines and weight stacks. Many of these are still useful tools to use for specific reasons, but they fail to address the way the human body functions in three dimensions and all directions.

The great Juan Carlos Santana, director of Institute of Human Performance in Boca Raton, Florida, teaches the best way to simplify human movement in developing effective conditioning and muscle building programs. Juan Carlos describes all of how we move as "The 4 Pillars of Human Motion."

He presents this very advanced concept in a very easy to understand manner that anyone can take home and use immediately to lose fat, build a sleek, muscular body, and prepare for the toughest of sports conditioning. Our tools include dumbbells, medicine balls, stability balls, resistance bands, bodyweight, and some exercise machines.

The exercises I will be giving you in the next few chapters are based on his remarkable system, so prepare to learn how easy it is to understand and improve your body at any age.

In functional training, the 4 pillars of human motion are:

1. Standing and Locomotion: Getting from one place to another, whether by walking, running, skipping, side shuffling, or agility drills.

2. Level Changes: Raising and lowering your center of mass, as in squats, lunges, going up and down stairs, or stepping on a box. These exercises will usually strengthen and firm your legs, hips and butt.

3. Pushing/Pulling: Anytime you push or pull against resistance. Every time you push the chest, shoulders and triceps get a workout. Conversely every time you perform a pulling action your lats, mid-traps, rhomboids, rear delt and biceps are working hard. When you do pushing/pulling exercises standing up then the entire body has a job to perform.

4. Rotation: Rotation exercises, which involve rotating your body, improve the muscles of your waist, sides and back.

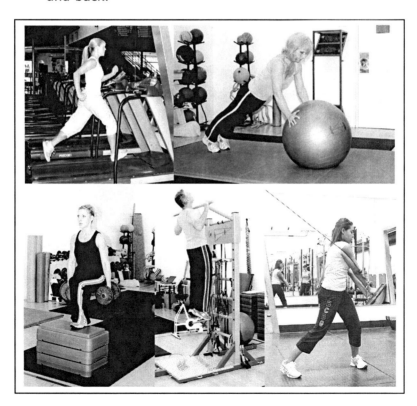

Your Exercise Program

Most Americans spend the majority of their days sitting. We sit at our desks, we sit at the movies, and we sit at restaurants. One of the most brilliant teachers of fitness and training, Juan Carlos Santana, teaches that the root of most of our physical problems today is the seated position which gives us tight, weak hip flexors, weak backs, weak butts, and ultimately leads to weight gain. In this chapter, I will show you how to counter the ill effects of sitting to your body.

Furthermore, the trunk is 360 degrees around the body, so just training your abs is an incomplete strategy. The trunk muscles rectus abdominus, internal and external obliques, transverse abdominus back extensors, multifidi, and rotatores must also be worked at least as much as the front of the body to provide strength, stability and proper movement. Therefore, many exercises that require you to stand give your abs a much better workout than endless sets of crunches.

In the next chapter, I will teach you how to do 45 seconds of posterior reach that can be performed anywhere, including in your office.

Warm Up Routine

A warm up routine does just that – warms up your muscles – as well as loosens your joints. Having muscles and joints that are prepared for your workout helps prevent injury while you exercise. I like to begin all of my workout sessions with two whole body sequences that prepare the muscles and central nervous system for the work ahead.

Wood Chops

Sequence one is called wood chops. It consists of straight up and down chopping motions to get our bodies out of the seated position. Then diagonal chops to each side to stretch and rotate the torso for active flexibility.

1. Wood Chops: Using a dumbbell or a medicine ball, reach with straight arms over your head to stretch the shoulders. Bend at the hips and bring the weight down between your bent legs. Repeat 10 times.

2. Diagonal Chops: Bring the weight from over head on one side and rotate diagonally, down to the other side. Pivot on the back foot.

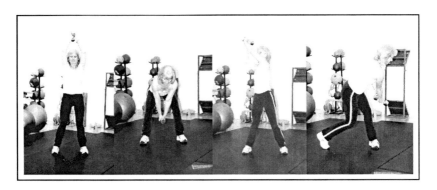

Gary's Matrix

The second is called "Gary's Matrix," designed by Gary Grey to provide total body preparation in all three planes of motion. It is composed of a pressing sequence (3 presses), a curling sequence (3), a lunging sequence (3 directions) and a lunge to press sequence.

Each exercise is performed alternately three times on each side. Choose light dumbbells between 5 and 15 pounds each.

Alternating Upright Press
Alternating Y Press

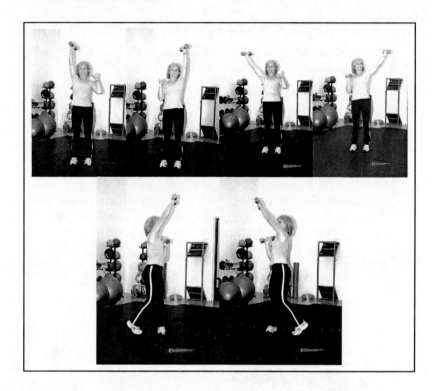

Alternating Curls

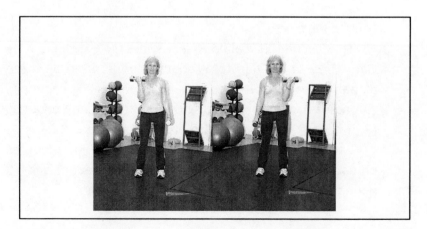

Alternating Upright Rows
Alternating Cross-Uppercuts

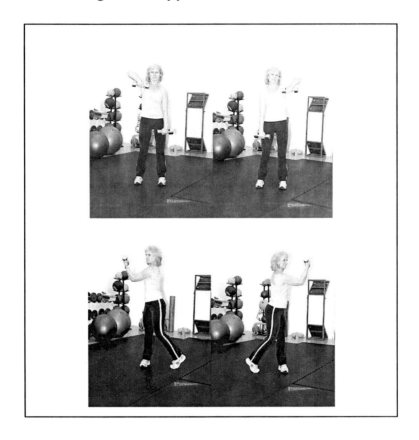

Tri-Planar Lunging

Following the upper body pushing and pulling sequences, we proceed to warming up the lower body in all three planes of motion with three on each side, alternating short lunge to the front with a reach, then reaching lunges to the sides and 135 degrees rotational reaching lunges.

Alternating Front Reaching Lunge

Take a short lunge forward and reach with the dumbbells to about the level of the top of your socks.

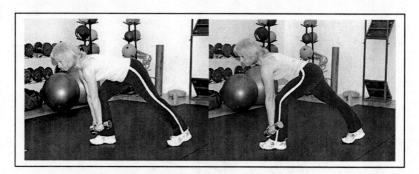

Alternating Side Reaching Lunge

Lunge to the side keeping the plant leg straight and both feet flat on the floor.

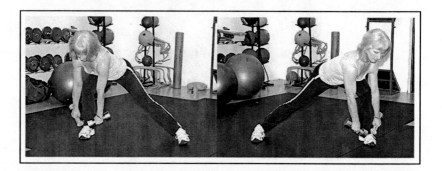

Alternating 135° Rotational Reaching Lunge

Lunge rotationally to the rear at a 135°

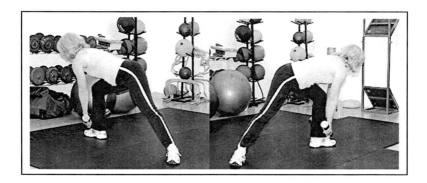

Lunge Sequence Press

Once you have completed the lunging sequence, repeat it with the addition of a press in between the lunges as shown. The side lunge to press is shown as an example.

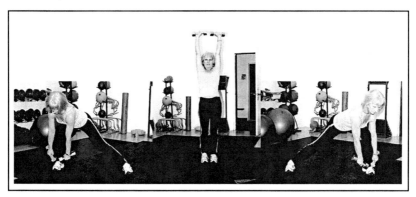

Level Changes Exercises

These exercises strengthen and tone primarily the leg muscles.

Resisted Step-up
- Grasp a challenging dumbbell in each hand.
- Place one foot on the step or bench.
- Keeping your back straight and tall and your shoulders back, step up onto the bench.
- Bring your working hip through at the top.
- Step down with control and keep your foot on the bench for your next repetition.
- Complete enough repetitions to make it exciting.
- Repeat with the other leg.

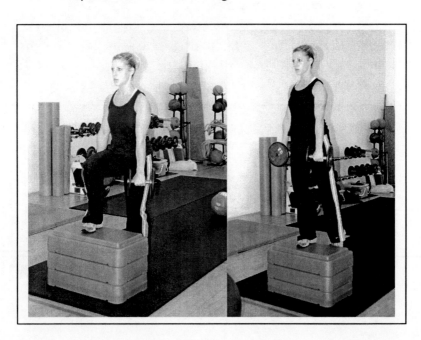

"Dan Ashley" Squats

These are Dan's favorite leg exercise, so we re-named them after him.

- Start in a seated position on the bench with your free leg extended.
- Push through the heel-arch of the working leg, keeping your free leg extended.
- Beginners can use a higher box to get started and then use lower as they get stronger.
- Advanced athletes can do away with the boxes and add resistance.

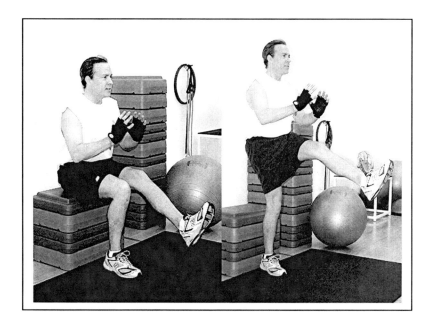

Back Squatting Mechanics
Preparation:

- Place your feet shoulder width apart or wider, slightly turned out or straight ahead. The wider and more turned out your feet, the more intense the exercise.
- Keep your waist braced front and back.

95

- Keep your chest up and out.
- Your eyes should be looking straight ahead.

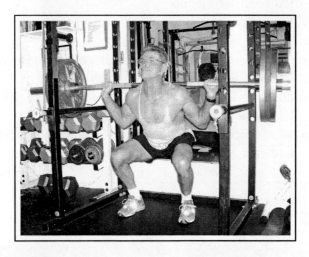

Descent:
- Butt goes back, back stays straight up with natural lordotic curve.
- The bar travels in a straight vertical line from the shoulders through the arch of the feet.
- With control lower the bar to your pain free range of motion to 90' or lower.

Ascent:
- Begin controlled lifting by tightening the glutes, contracting the quadriceps and exhaling on the way up. Be sure that your shoulders are rising at the same speed as your hips.
- Rise to a soft knee without locking.

Finishing:
- Walk the bar all the way in until it touches the backstop.
- Remove Plates from the bar when finished.

Anterior Reach and Single Leg Squat

The anterior reach is the ultimate in functional leg exercises that will enhance your running stride, your ability to stabilize on one leg and change direction. Begin by balancing on a single leg and reach toward a given target with your opposite hand.

Start with 5 reps on each side and progress to 15 on each side. Use only the speed that you can control.

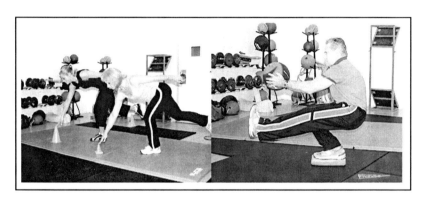

Triple Threats: My Favorite "Back of Legs" Exercise

This exercise will not only firm up the back of your legs like no other, but it will also enhance stride mechanics and improve running stride length.

Begin with sets of 5/5/5 with two legs then increase reps by 1/1/1 each week until you can perform 15/15/15 in perfect form for three sets. After getting good at 15's, try the advanced progression by performing them using one leg at a time.

When you go to one leg, begin with 5/5/5 again and progress by adding 1/1/1 per week until at 15's you have developed hamstrings of steel in 20 weeks.

1. Begin triple threats supine with the ball under the heels of your feet.
2. Press your heels downward very hard with straight legs and toes together. The work being done by your hamstrings, glutes and back muscles will cause your hips to rise. Don't allow your butt to hit the ground for the rest of the exercise.
3. While keeping your hips extended, curl the ball in toward your butt by contracting your hamstrings and calf muscles. Your hips should rise even higher when you do it correctly.
4. Without letting your hips hit the floor, walk the ball out until only the balls of your feet are in contact with the edge of the ball. Repeat the hip lift again, but now your are on your toes and it is like you added a calf raise to the hip lift. You will feel a huge burn in your hammies by the time you finish this part of the set.

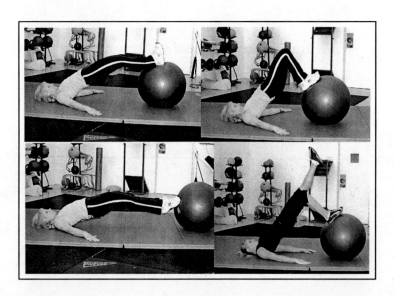

Pushing Exercises

All pushing exercises work the chest, shoulders and triceps. When you pull the lats (back muscles), rear delts, and biceps get involved. When you do a pushing or pulling exercise while standing, the entire core muscles are required to stabilize the body, as well.

Stability Ball Dumbbell Bench Press
- Begin by stabilizing yourself on a stability ball with your shoulders across the top center as shown.
- Raise and lower the dumbbells with control.
- You can also alternate the presses one arm at a time.

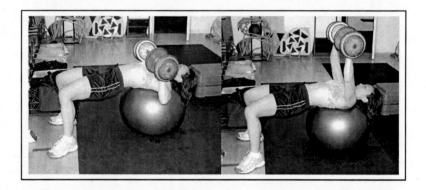

Standing Press Using Resistance Bands
Any kind of standing press with a cable-pulley or band will challenge more body parts and increase the metabolic cost. When using a staggered stance, this type of pressing motion also engages the front core musculature and the glute/ham extensors of the rear leg and hip.

- You can make the exercise more interesting by alternating the press and rotating at the hip and oblique muscles.
- Be sure to try single arm pushes as well.

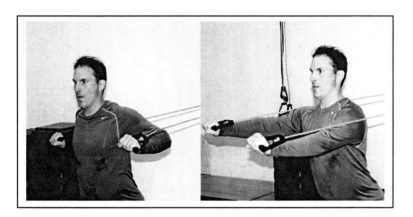

Stability Ball Push-Up

This exercise targets the chest, front shoulder, triceps, abs, hips, quadriceps and ankles.

- Begin with your torso on the ball and your hand facing down on the ball as shown.
- Push up while bracing the core and keeping your butt tucked in.
- You can make the exercise very easy just by placing the ball higher on steps or a chair.
- Elevating your feet or going to one hand push-ups will challenge most advanced athletes.

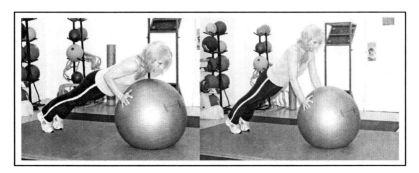

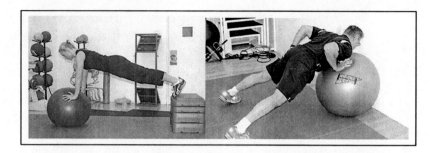

Bench Press

- Lying on a bench with your nose under the bar, grasp the barbell with a slightly wider than shoulders grip.
- Bring the bar up and over your chest before lowering with a controlled speed to nipple level.
- Push the bar up to straight arm position.
- Rack the weight securely when finished.
- This works the chest, front of the shoulders, and back of your arms.

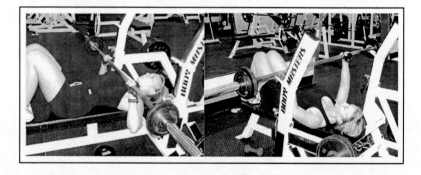

Dumbbell Incline Bench Press

This exercise is known for filling in the upper pectoral muscles of the chest.

- From the starting position, hold the weights in line with your upper chest and your forearms perpendicular to the floor.
- Raise the dumbbells up and slightly toward each other without clanging them at the top.
- Lower the dumbbells with control and repeat for your given amount of reps with the weight used.

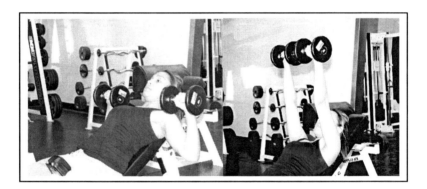

Pulling Exercises

Rope Pulls

1. Begin by anchoring your feet against a wall.
2. Grip the rope tightly, then lower yourself to put the lats on stretch. Avoid sagging in your middle by keeping your body stiff.
3. With your chest up and out, pull up to starting position. Be sure to squeeze your shoulder blades together to enhance your benefits from the exercise.
4. You can also do this exercise with a jungle gym apparatus as shown below.

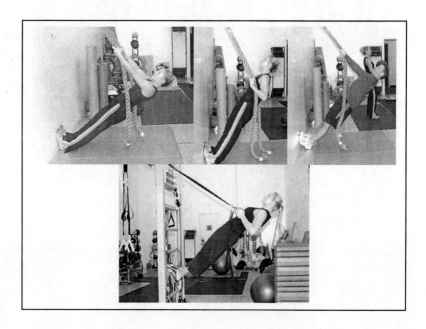

Lat Pull-Downs/Chin-Ups

1. On a pull-down machine grip the bar tightly with a wider than shoulders grip.
2. Pull your shoulders back first to retract the scapula, then bend the elbows and keep pulling until the bar touches your upper chest. It should feel like you are squeezing your shoulder blades together.
3. With control bring the bar back to the starting position.
4. Advanced athletes can do chin-ups on a bar with body weight before adding a weighted vest or dumbbells for extra resistance.

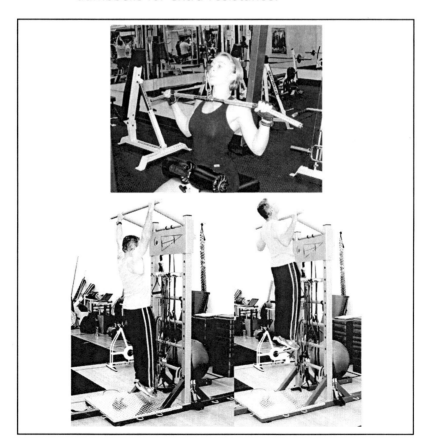

Various Cable Rows

I like to use a staggered stance for standing rowing exercises. These are my favorite for working not only the back pulling muscles but also the front supporting leg and lower back muscles isometrically.

Cable row exercise descriptions:

1. After selecting a challenging weight, grasp the handle of the cable using a staggered stance.
2. The lower your stance, the more work your front leg will have to do to resist being pulled forward.
3. Brace your core and pull the cable from an extended to a flexed arm, position.
4. Repeat on the opposite side.

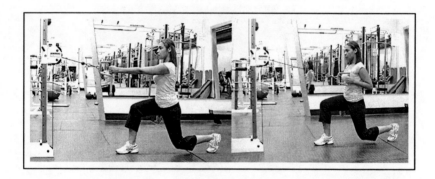

Rotation and Core Exercises

Since 90 percent of our muscles lay diagonally throughout our bodies, our bodies indicate that we are designed to rotate. Almost everything we do requires rotation.

Cable or Medicine Ball Chops
You cannot beat rotational chops for conditioning your core 360 degrees front, back and sides.

High-to-Low Chops
1. With a cable or stretch band mounted above your head, stand with your feet perpendicular to the wire or band.
2. Grasp the handle with both hands then with stiff arms, rotate diagonally down and across your body towards your opposite knee. You can also pivot on your back foot as you rotate when you become advanced.
3. Control the return to starting position and make sure you get a good stretch in your obliques at the top before repeating.

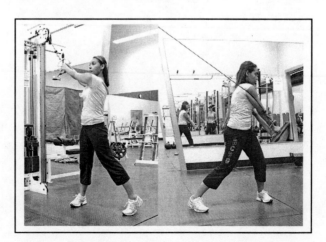

Low-to-High Chops
1. Begin by reversing the cable or band to a low setting and start with the cable or band handle just past your knee, near the stripe in your pants. Knees are bent. You can also use a dumbbell.
2. Raise the cable up and diagonally across your body while simultaneously extending your knees and back hip. Pivot the back foot as you rotate.

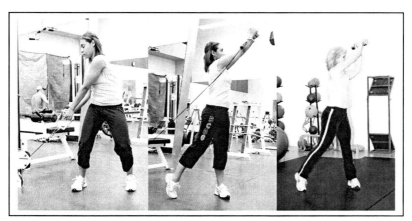

Side Chops
1. Place the cable or band handle a little below shoulder level.
2. Rotate side to side.
3. A variation is to use a very heavy band or resistance and use a short and quick 10-2 o'clock motion

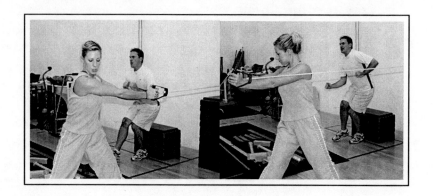

Rotational V-Ups

From a seated position on a mat or pad, rotate a medicine ball side to side with stiff arms as shown. Be sure to keep your arms locked and as straight as possible. This works the rectus abdominus, internal and external obliques and hip flexors.

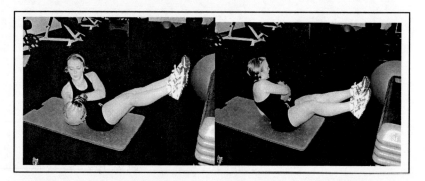

Medicine-Ball Wall Slam

From a supine position on the mat with arms extended behind you, explosively sit up as you toss the medicine ball against the wall. Be sure to keep the ball away from your face as you catch it and repeat. If you miss the ball you risk a broken nose or other facial injury.

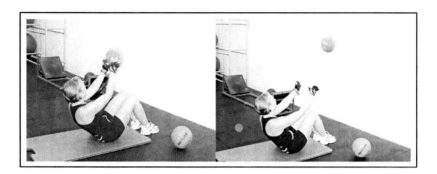

Floor or Ball Crunches

Begin in a supine position on floor or ball then flex your trunk while keeping the hips up. You can add resistance with a band, cable, medicine ball or weight plate.

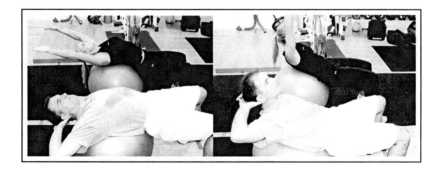

Circuit Training:
Putting the Exercises Together

How to Create Your Own Effective Program

I am training you the same way I train my clients and myself. You can make your circuits using as little as 3 to as many as 12 or more exercises in a row, blending the 4 pillars of human motion to challenge and improve your entire body.

Listed below are two ways that I accomplish this. One is by using two separate circuits of 4 exercises of three rounds each. The other is the one I use in my "Give Fat the Boot Camp" classes where 12 exercises are linked with each exercise performed for 40 seconds with a 20-second transition time to get to the next exercise and recover your breath a little. Repeat each circuit 3 times in this option. Follow these types of strength training with some cardio intervals, and your body will be looking good and stoked for fat loss.

Four-Exercise Circuit

Now that you are familiar with the individual exercises, it's easy to create your program.
1. For circuit one, pick one exercise representing each of the four pillars of human movement. Then choose four different exercises from each pillar for circuit two.
2. Perform each set of the exercises from circuit 1 for 8-12 repetitions in perfect form. Your tempo should be 4 seconds to lower the weight, and 1 second to raise it. (4-0-1)

3. Repeat circuit one 3-5 times before moving on the circuit 2 which you can also do for 3-5 sets.
4. Finish with 20 minutes of steady state cardio for health.

You can be very creative with your exercise selections once you get used to using the four pillars of human motion approach to selecting which exercises to use. Here is and example.

Circuit 1	Circuit 2
bench step-up	triple threats
bench press	med-ball push-up
lat pull	1-arm row
high-to-low chops	med-ball wall slams

Or set it up like this in your training log:

Squat		/	/	/	
Stability Ball Push-up		/	/	/	
Chin-ups		/	/	/	
Low to High Chops		/	/	/	
Triple threats		/	/	/	
One arm DB row		/	/	/	
DB Incline Press		/	/	/	
SB Back extensions		/	/	/	

Twelve-Exercise Circuit

Example: Perform each exercise for 40 seconds, then allow a 15- 20 second transition time to get to the next exercise and to take a few breaths. A similar protocol with some more challenging exercises is featured on my *Hotel Room Boot Camp* DVD. Repeat the circuit 3 times. Rest for 1 minute between each circuit.

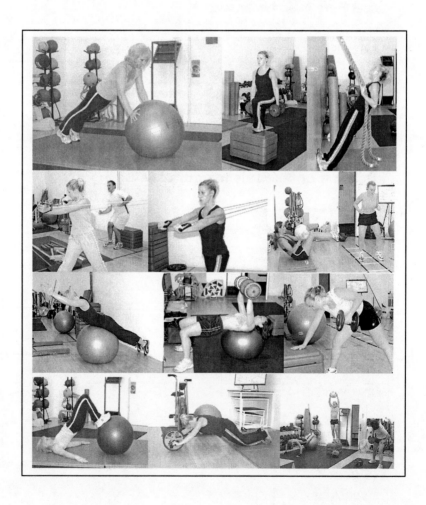

Post-Workout Recovery

I'm going to be very clear on this principle. Without sufficient recovery, you will never achieve your maximum potential for weight loss, muscle gain or athletic ability. Post-workout recovery strategies include a form of self massage known as bio-foam rollouts, stretching, REST, and of course a supportive nutrition plan.

Bio-foam Roller Work

The first thing to do following a tough exercise session is to roll out the knots in your muscles. In the past, it was said that stretching after a workout was essential. Since then we have found out that if you keep stretching a knot, it just gets tighter and tighter.

When you learn how to do use the bio-foam roller for self massage, your muscles, joints, ligaments and tendons will thank you. You will enjoy improved tissue quality, flexibility and reduced muscle soreness. It's a little tricky to learn how to position your body on the rollers but once you get it then a cheap effective deep tissue massage is yours in minutes. Following the roll-outs, stretching will be much more effective.

Lower Body Rollouts
Iliotibial Band, Front Quadriceps, Medial Thigh

Position yourself as shown on the roller for IT band roll. Use your arms and supporting leg to control the pressure on the part that you are rolling. Roll from just above the knee joint to the hip 6-10 times.

For the front quadriceps, place your free leg outside of the roller as shown in the second photo. Roll from the top of the knee to the hip.

It's a little tricky to get the position for rolling over the inside leg muscles but with a little practice it will become more natural. Take a four point stance, turn out your rolling leg to position the inside of the thigh against the roller, then roll from just above the knee over the vastus medialis and inside of thigh.

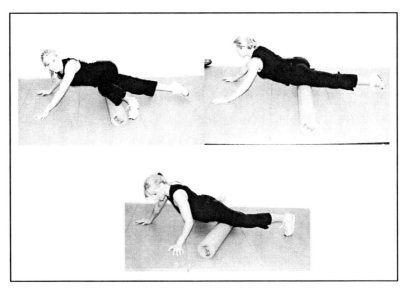

Calf, Hamstrings, Glutes

For your calf muscles, sit down with your supporting leg outside the roller and your hands placed behind you. Place your calf on the roller and roll from just below the knee joint to the bottom of your calf. You can also turn your leg out and roll over the outside portion of your calf muscle.

Reposition yourself so that the roller is just below your glutes, then roll down to just above your knee to get the back of your thighs.

Another tricky position is to sit somewhat side-saddle on the roller, place your front foot above your supporting leg's knee as shown and gently roll a few inches at a time across your glute muscles. These will be very uncomfortable at first which just shows how much you need to do it regularly. The discomfort will diminish as your muscle tissue quality improves.

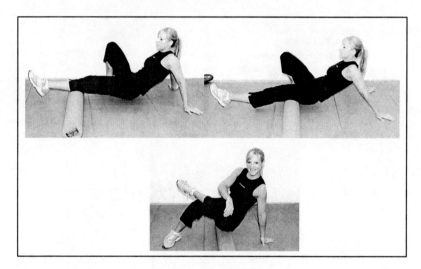

Upper Body Rollouts
Thoracic Spine, and Lat Roll

These will feel real good if you do them carefully. Place the roller just below your scapulae, keeping your butt on the floor for now. Slowly and with control, reach back and extend your arms.

Repeat the process three times moving up the spine one vertebra at a time. Then fold your arms in front of your body and roll over the entire thoracic spine area.

To massage your lats, turn sideways as shown and gently at first, roll over your big latissimus muscles. These may also be very uncomfortable so you can use your supporting hand on the roller to adjust the pressure to make it bearable until you improve. Remember, the more it hurts with these rollouts, the more crucial it is that you do them.

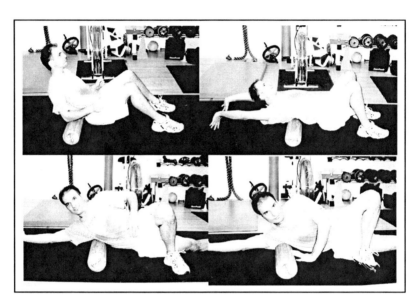

Static Stretches

Static stretches are performed after your workout with active flexibility taking preference in your warm-up and strength training activities. Because static stretches isolate specific muscles, they are the most beneficial type of stretch.

Keep in mind that safe and effective stretches are done only to a feeling of slight tightness or discomfort. Never stretch to a position that is painful. Hold your pain free stretch for 20-30 seconds.

Seated Hamstring Stretch

Wrap the rope around the middle of your foot and grasp the rope firmly. Keep your back stiff and straight as you lean forward from the waist until you feel a slightly uncomfortable pull in the back of your legs.

Hold for 20-30 seconds, then switch to the other leg. Avoid rounding your back – this will take the stretch off your targeted hamstrings.

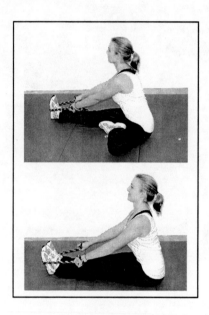

Seated Double Hamstring Stretch

Wrap the rope around both feet and grasp the rope firmly. Keep your back stiff and straight as you lean forward from the waist until you feel the pull in back of both legs.

Hold for 20-30 seconds. Avoid rounding the back as this will take the stretch off your targeted hamstrings.

Supine Hamstring Rope Stretch

Lie supine on the mat. Wrap the rope around your foot. While keeping the opposite leg on the floor, pull the rope until you feel a nice pull in the back of your leg and hold for 20-30 seconds. Switch legs. Do not allow your hip to come off the mat.

You can also actively stretch by holding for two seconds, relaxing for two and repeating.

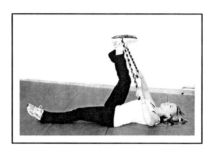

Supine Hip Stretch

With the rope wrapped around your left foot, hold the rope in your right hand and bring your leg across your body as shown. Pull up until a mild stretch is felt in the hamstrings and left hip. Allow gravity to assist in stretching the hip.

Hold for 20-30 seconds or apply the previously described active stretching technique. Switch sides.

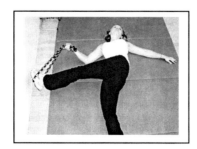

Bent Knee Hip Stretch

To intensify the stretch in your left hip, you can bend your knee and bring your arm across your upper leg to help stretch your glutes and hips.

Be sure to keep your opposite shoulder on the mat. Switch legs.

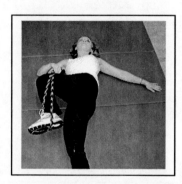

Prone Quad and Hip Flexor Stretch

Double wrap the rope around your foot and gently pull on the rope as shown until you feel the stretch in front of your leg and hip.

You can intensify the stretch by pushing your hip into the floor as you hold the stretch for 20-30 seconds. Switch legs.

Avoid severely arching the back in order to prevent scrunching your posterior spinal processes – if it hurts, do not do it.

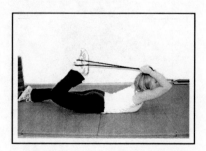

Stability Ball Piriformis and Glute Stretch

Lying supine on the mat, place your left foot on the top of the ball and cross your right leg above the left knee as shown. When you toll the ball close to the body you will feel a delicious stretch in the target areas.

Hold for 20-30 seconds then switch legs.

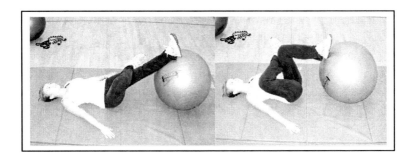

Standing Shoulder Stretch

Grasp the rope a little wider than shoulder width and reach back as far as you can to stretch the front of your shoulders. Avoid pushing your head forward as you reach back. Keep your neck relaxed

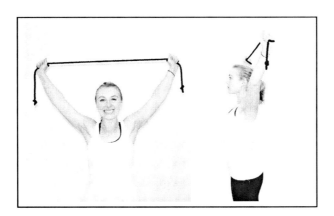

Standing Chest and Shoulder Stretch

Grasp the rope a little wider so that you can lower it behind your chest. This should feel awesome in the chest area. Keep your neck relaxed and your head back.

Bringing the rope lower will stretch the chest and shoulders even more intensely and improve your flexibility in the shoulder joint area.

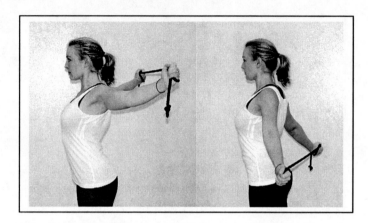

Side Stretch – Left and Right

This stretch will loosen up your internal and external obloquies as well as your lats and posterior shoulder joint.

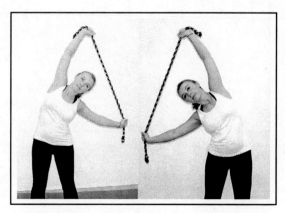

Triceps Stretch

This is a good stretch after a hard arm workout to maintain flexibility in the back of the arm and front/lower area of the shoulder joint.

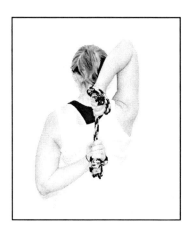

Home Exercise Training Tips

Not everyone can or wants to use a gym to meet their fitness goals. If you life too far away from a gym, are on the road a lot, or would rather just work out at home, this chapter gives you the home training strategies you need to succeed on your own. Learn how to adhere to a home exercise program, use the most effective exercises, get the best use of your treadmill, and more.

With Minimal Inexpensive Exercise Equipment

Using resistance bands, bodyweight, stability balls, you can avoid the gym, and still enjoy challenging workouts that lead to dramatic positive changes for your body.

A Complete Home or Hotel Workout

When you want to get a muscle preserving and calorie burning workout at home or while traveling, all you will need is a J.C. Traveler band and your own body.

The following exercises can be done as a 12 station circuit or broken up into three sets of a four exercise quadplex.

For example pick 4 exercises that include a push, pull, level change and core. Perform each exercise in a circuit for 40 seconds each. Repeat three times, then pick 4 more exercises that are different and do the same thing.

When using a 12 exercise circuit, like the one illustrated, be sure to sequence the exercises with a good mix of the four pillars. Perform each exercise for

40 seconds with a 20 second transition time before going to the next one. Repeat the circuit three times.

When using a JC Traveler band, be sure to mount it in the inside part of the door with the hinges on the other side. This will provide the most secure fastening of the band with less risk of it coming out and injuring you.

Be sure to close the door tight. Also make sure that the nubby part of the band is all the way in and give it a good tug before moving on to the exercises.

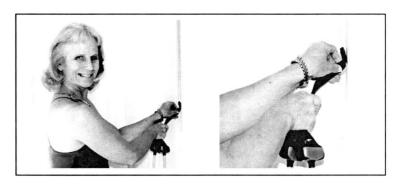

The Exercises

Now that you know about the four pillars of human movement we can apply this to create a challenging and fun workout that takes very little time out of your vacation or business travel.

Pushes

1. Standing Two-Arm Press: Take a good staggered stance with your back leg straight and stiff. Tighten up your back glute cheek and stand straight and tall to engage your abs. Press forward to a straight arm and return slowly to a count of 4. This exercise works the chest muscles, triceps and front shoulder

muscles primarily. It also challenges the stabilizers in the abs and back glute.

2. Incline Band Press: Mount the band in the lowest part of the door jamb. Use the same staggered stance as above and push at a 45 degree angle instead of straight ahead. This emphasizes the upper part of the chest muscles as well as those listed above.

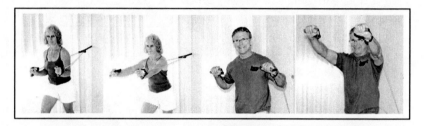

3. Single Arm Band Press: Take the staggered stance, but this time bend your back leg and put the weight on the ball of the back foot. This will actively stretch your calves as well as make them and your ankles work. Your inner and external obliques will also work harder to resist rotation. Keep your hips facing toward the front.

4. Low Rotational Punch: Attach the rope high in the doorjamb and bend over in a staggered stance. Rotate your torso to initiate the arm extension to give your core muscles a good burn while working your chest and arms.

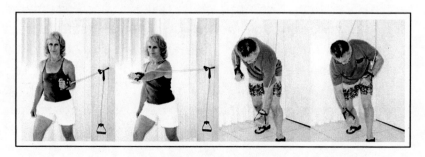

5. Chair Push-ups: Beginners can place their hands on the chair. Advanced can place feet or one foot on the chair. Be sure to keep the ankles, knees, hips, abs and back absolutely still and stable while raising and lowering.

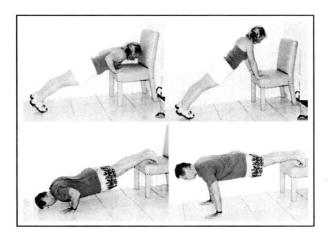

Pulls

For lat pull place the band in the top part of the doorjamb. Use the staggered stance or one knee on the floor. Pull the band toward you with your hands in a neutral position. Be sure to bring the elbows back as far as possible while retracting the scapulae and maintaining an erect posture.

1. Standing Two-Arm Row: Place the band in a shoulder height area of the doorjamb. Take a very low staggered stance in order to make your front leg work harder to resist being pulled forward. Keep your back straight and pull back as far as possible as above.

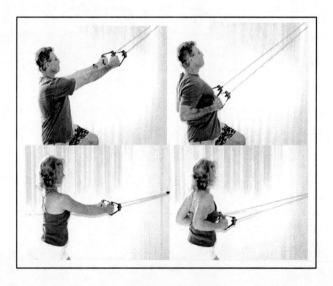

2. A one arm pull requires resisting rotation in the transverse plane so your obliques will be engaged as well as the supporting stance leg. This is my favorite rowing exercise.

3. Biceps Curl: Step on the webbed part of a short JC Traveler Band and with your arms tucked firmly to your sides, curl the handles up against the resistance

to challenge and grow bigger bicep muscles. Be sure to control the lowering of the band to make the muscle work harder.

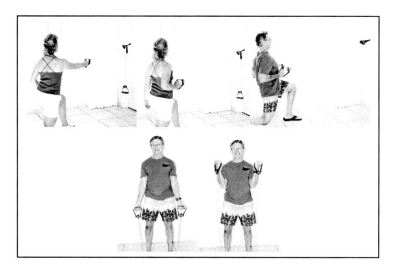

Level Changes

1. Single Leg Squat Reach: Balance on one leg while reaching for the sunblock bottle with the opposite hand.

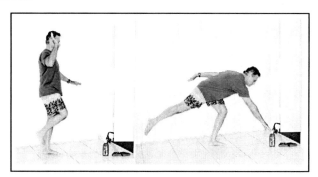

2. Single Leg Chair Squat: Balance on one leg while extending the other in front. With control, sit back from the hip until your seat barely touches the chair.

Push down into the floor with your heel and stand up. Repeat on opposite leg.

3. Resisted Single Leg Squat Reach: Same as 1 but with band resistance.

4. Single Leg Front Squat: Same as chair squat without the chair (very advanced).

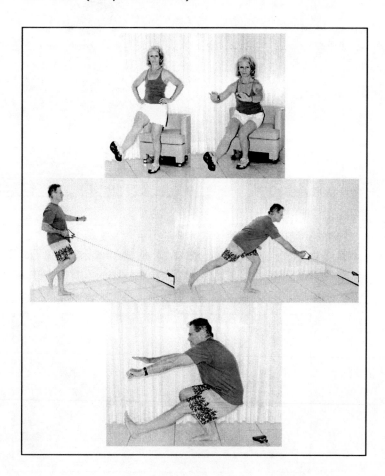

Core and Abs

1. High to Low Chops: Insert the band into the uppermost part of the door jamb and rotate the body diagonally, bringing the handles down and across the front of your body. Make sure that as you rotate, you keep your arms only slightly bent and the band stays in the groove between your elbow and shoulder.

2. Leg Lowers: Lie flat on your back with your feet up and legs straight. Keep your back absolutely flat on the floor while lowering your legs very slowly. Lower only as far as you can while keeping your back from arching. Stop lowering and hold for 30 seconds at this point. As you get stronger you will be able to lower your legs closer to the floor.

3. Low to High Chops: With the band in the lowest part of the doorjamb, rotate the band diagonally up while keeping a naturally straight back. Pivot on the back foot.

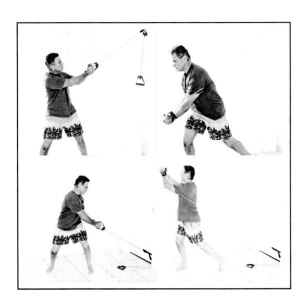

4. Planks: Lie prone on a towel as if you are on the beach reading a book. Dig your toes into the floor; tighten your legs, hips, abs and shoulders. Hold as long as you can from 5- 60 seconds.

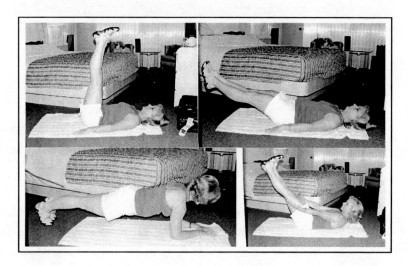

Home Treadmills, Elliptical Machines, and Exercise Bikes

If you want to buy a treadmill, get the best treadmill that you can afford. A five thousand dollar treadmill that lasts for fifteen years is less expensive than a three thousand dollar treadmill that lasts for two years or less.

Personally, I like *Sports-Art* and *Free Motion* treadmills. Be sure you get one with a suspended deck for shock absorption. Also, look for a belt that is wide and long enough for you to be comfortable running.

Precor makes some of the best ellipticals. Again, bargain prices often are not a good deal.

Schwinn Airdyne is one of the best home aerobic pieces that you can get for the price. New ones are

134

about $700 dollars and can be used safely for intense fat loss workouts. Remember to ignore what every piece of cardio equipment says about the fat burning zone and use my metabolism increasing interval protocols.

Supportive Nutrition

Do you feel like you are stuck in a rut with your eating plan? Same thing day in and day out-chicken-chicken-chicken, tuna-tuna-tuna. Or maybe you simply do not have an eating plan. In this chapter, you will learn what to eat, what to avoid, and how to stimulate your fat loss success with the right food choices.

I use the term supportive nutrition to describe a lifestyle of better choices for healthy eating rather than endlessly chasing after a diet that will not work. Supportive nutrition will provide you with plenty of energy for your daily life and exercise and with all you need to successfully develop muscle and reduce fat on your body. When the right nutrition becomes part of your life, you can achieve dramatic results even if you have experienced failure with ineffective strategies in the past.

I also have mentioned many times that the main reason that people have failed to achieve the fitness and weight loss results that they desire from other programs is because they have been mislead. Usually, the easiest way to spot a defective program is to notice that the words "quick and easy" are included in the pitch.

Supportive nutrition consists of a balanced program of frequent eating, including lean sources of protein, starchy carbohydrates (carbs), and fibrous carbohydrates. Lean protein sources include lean meat, eggs, chicken, turkey, nuts, seeds, and fish. Starchy carbs include potatoes, brown rice, whole grain pastas, and whole grain breads. Fibrous carbs are the greens in a salad, green beans, broccoli, asparagus, and other vegetables.

Portion sizes can follow simple guidelines like a protein source being the size of a deck of cards. The starchy and fibrous carbs should measure about a cup each.

Diets that require you to eat only special foods do more for the financial state of the founder than for the health condition of the dieter. They also make you dependent upon them by failing to allow you to think for yourself. Supportive nutrition works because it teaches you to make modifications in your lifestyle and to develop supportive habits that are simple to implement and satisfying to live with. The concept of "cheat days" and speeding up your metabolism allows you to be less than perfect and still achieve optimal results. If you learn what you need your meals to consist of in terms of nutrients (proteins, carbs, and fats), then you can create any meals you want. Just be sure to avoid saturated fats and sugar.

Keep in mind that, if you want a healthy, permanent body transformation, you must apply the synergy of strength training, moderate cardiovascular training, and supportive nutrition.

Calories

Many diets require dieters to count calories, but how many calories should you really be counting to be healthy, and what is a calorie, anyway?

A calorie is a unit of food energy. In order to determine how much energy you need to provide for your body through what you eat, you need to use a little math. By adding your metabolic rate, the energy you expend during physical activity, and the thermic effect of the food you eat, you can determine how much energy your body uses, or how many calories your body needs in a day. Your basal metabolic rate (BMR) is how much energy you burn while at rest – how much energy your organs and nervous system use without taking into account the energy burned by your deliberate physical activity. The functions of your body account for about 70 percent of the calories you burn in a day. The Harris-Benedict formula, which determines your BMR based on your body weight is below:

For Men: BMR =
66 + (13.7 x weight in kg) + (5 x height in cm) - (6.8 x age in years)

For Women: BMR =
655 + (9.6 x weight in kg) + (1.8 x height in cm) - (4.7 x age in years)

Keep in mind that 1 inch equals 2.54 cm and 1 kilogram is 2.2 pounds.

Your level of physical activity is the next element in determining how many calories you need to eat each day. This aspect of your body's use of calories accounts from approximately 20 to 30 percent of the calories you burn each day.

In order to determine this number, you must calculate your level of activity multiplied by your BMR to determine how many calories you burn due to physical activity each day.

Sedentary (little or no exercise)
= BMR x 1.2

Lightly Active (light exercise 1-3 days a week)
= BMR x 1.375

Most people will fall into the first two categories unless they are professional athletes or work hard physical labor. Even if you do an hour of exercise every day it still leaves 23 light hours.

Moderately Active (moderate exercise 3-5 days a week)
= BMR x 1.55

Very Active (hard exercise 6-7 days a week)
= BMR x 1.725

Extremely Active (hard daily exercise and a physically demanding job or twice a day athletic training)
= BMR x 1.9

Your answer is the total number of calories you need to maintain your current weight. The thermic effect of digesting foods is not included in the calories calculated because your brain counts what is ingested. This will be useful in helping to create your caloric deficit and over time will assist in fat loss.

Now that you have done all the separate equations, you can determine your total daily need for calories:

BMR Calories + Activity Calories

Using what you have learned here, you can determine how many calories you should eat each day. As your lean body mass raises and your energy expenditure during activity raises, you will want to adjust your calorie intake. Each pound of fat equals 3,500 calories, meaning to lose 3,500 calories, you need to eat 3,500 fewer calories (within the healthy parameters discussed in this book) or spend 3,500 calories more while maintaining the same amount of calorie intake you currently have.

Pre-Packaged, Processed Foods

"You are what you eat" is a sort of silly phrase, but there is quite a bit of accuracy to it nonetheless. If you eat processed foods, instead of fresh, healthy foods, your body will suffer from the low quality of food you are giving it. We often think of our food in terms of convenience and taste, but our food thinks of our food in terms of nutrition and energy potential. Processed food, by definition, are unnatural, providing little if any nutritional resources for your very natural body to utilize. You body cannot properly digest the preservatives, chemicals, and additives of processed foods and your body received only minimal nutrients in these harmful foods. Fresh foods, on the other hand, make all the difference in the efficiency and well-being of your body's many systems.

The Importance of Protein

Your body is composed of millions of elements and systems, but its main component is protein; your body needs protein to build and repair your cells, muscles, and tissue. You are not capable of producing your own essential amino acids, which are vital to most aspects of life, meaning you have to introduce them into your body

140

through the foods you eat. Proteins are composed of amino acids, providing your body one of its most essential elements through the lean healthy sources of protein you should be giving it. These amino acids are vital to your wellbeing, regenerating your tissue, cells, and muscles.

As an athlete, you need to utilize the benefits of high levels of protein in your diet. If your body is properly supplied the protein it needs through your diet, you are making sure that you provide your body with the most efficient and effective energy and repair system it can maintain. With enough protein in your diet, your body can continue to grow, heal, and repair itself, allowing you to advance in your training.

Furthermore, in working toward your ideal body, you will want to know that protein is more difficult for your body to metabolize, meaning that you increase your metabolism each time you eat protein. In fact, almost one third of the calories you ingest by eating high-protein foods are burned just by eating the food. All of my most respected experts recommend 1 gram per pound of bodyweight.

Thermogenesis

One of the most interesting aspects of high-protein foods is its stimulation of thermogenesis. Thermogenesis is the process that your body uses to create heat within your body. The most common forms of thermogenesis are in hibernating, small children, and all mammals in freezing weather, but it also occurs after every time you eat. Thermogenesis burns a lot of energy stored in your fat cells, meaning it boosts your metabolism each time you eat.

Obviously, this does not mean that sitting at your desk all day with a bad of potato chips and a 44 ounce soda is going to up your metabolism and burn your excess fat. Protein is food of choice for stimulating thermogenesis in your body. Because protein requires your body to expend more energy than most foods for your body to be able to digest it, protein stimulates the thermogenic effect more than other foods.

If you maintain a diet that promotes keeping your body's energy balance, such as eating six small meals a day, and a diet that includes high-protein foods, you can continuously activate thermogenesis in your body, constantly boosting your metabolism. Also, by eating six times a day instead of three, you trigger our thermogenesis six times a day instead of just three.

If you are not eating five to six thermic meals of the proper portions of lean protein, complex starchy carb, and fibrous carb foods, then you will find it difficult to achieve that body of your dreams.

Carbohydrates

Carbohydrates do not raise your metabolism as much as protein, but they do provide your body with energy. Approximately 7-10% of calories from carbohydrates are burned during the eating process. Carbs are in all plant foods and in some dairy foods and are composed of sugar molecules. When you eat carbs, your body does not use them to repair your body as it does proteins; it converts the carbs into glucose, which provides your cells with energy. Eating food that gives you energy is a very important part of your diet, but eating excess carbs will lead to fat storage. Your body will convert the extra glucose to triglycerides and store it in fat cells.

Although carbs have gotten a really bad name in the media in the past few years, removing carbs from your diet altogether would be an extremely unhealthy act, virtually depriving your body of the main ingredient it needs for energy production.

There are two types of carbohydrates. Simple carbs, which are sometimes referred to as simple sugars, are found in dairy products, fruits, and candy and sweets. They are made up of sugar and are generally known as the "bad" carbs due to their extremely low nutritional value and high calorie counts. Complex carbohydrates, however, although they are made of sugar as well, are starches and fibers that are full of vitamins, minerals, nutrients, and fiber, earning them the name "good" carbs. Complex carbs are found in legumes, starchy vegetables, and whole grains.

Your body converts the carbohydrates you eat into glucose, which is the sugar in your bloods that your body uses for energy or stores in fat cells to potentially burn later for energy. Your glycemic response to foods is a measurement of how quickly your body breaks down those carbohydrates in the energy-producing process.

If your body breaks down a particular food very quickly, the glucose enters your blood very quickly and rapidly raises your blood sugar level. A sharp increase in your blood sugar level is the spike and drop in energy levels mentioned above. This process is not only frustrating when trying to sustain high energy levels, but is unhealthy as well.

If a foods glycemic index is high, eating it will cause you to experience this energy cycle, but if the glycemic index is low, you can avoid this annoying and unhealthy process. The change in your blood sugar level is much less dramatic when you eat foods that rank low on the glycemic index. You can probably guess through your own experiences which foods rank high and low on this index. White bread, potatoes, and junk foods in general have high glycemic index and whole grains and green vegetables have low indexes.

In addition to eating foods that have good glycemic indexes, eating frequent, small meals each day help to keep your blood sugar level steady, avoiding spikes and pits in your energy levels as well as avoiding cravings for carbohydrates.

In order to avoid the bad carbs and to be sure to include the good carbs in your diet, just look for vegetables that come out of the ground, and whole grain products like whole wheat bread, brown rice and whole grain pastas. Be sure to inspect labels carefully.

"But Coach, isn't fruit healthy?"

Yes, fruit is very healthy and if fat loss is your goal I recommend that you eat it in the presence of a lean protein, since the body will then recognize a reduced *glycemic load* of the meal. For example, if you ate blueberries with Trader Joe's Non-fat Greek Style Yogurt, you would have a nutritious snack instead of an insulin spiking event.

Fats

Obviously, if you are reading this book and implementing my fitness plan in your life, you want to get rid of your excess fat. However, you may not realize that fat is a vital part of your diet. Your body uses fat for all sorts of extremely important functions. Important vitamins, such as vitamins A, D, E, and K are fat-soluble

– your body needs essential fatty acids to digest, absorb, and utilize them. Fat protects your body's organs, helps your body to maintain your body temperature, and is even essential to skin and hair health.

Similar to carbohydrates, fats can be divided into good and bad categories. Some fats are essential to your health – you must eat foods with these fats because your body cannot produce them on its own. Other fats are very unhealthy because your body has no use for them and cannot process them effectively, leading to clogged arteries and many other common health problems.

Good fats include monounsaturated fats and polyunsaturated fats. Both these fats lower your body cholesterol, and monounsaturated fats actually raise your good cholesterol. I take three flax oil gel-capsules every morning with my breakfast. I believe that my skin and joints have been thanking me since I began taking them.

Saturated fats and trans fats, however, are extremely unhealthy and should be avoided. Saturated fat raises your bad cholesterol, and trans fat, which is an unnatural invention to help process foods that are bound for commercial packaging, holds absolutely no nutritional value and cannot be used by your body for anything.

Keeping this information in mind as you plan your meals is extremely important to your health. Try not to use oils such as coconut, vegetable, and palm when you cook because these contain large amounts of saturated and trans fats. Use canola, olive, and flax seed oil for your cooking because these contain large amounts of monounsaturated fats and small amounts of saturated fats.

In general, do not eat commercially packaged foods. As mentioned, they are too full of chemicals and too deprived of nutrients to even be considered as part of a healthy diet. Low fat dairy and lean meats are the way to go when you are preparing meals. Train yourself to check the nutrition labels and take heed of saturated fat and trans fat levels.

Fiber

Soluble fiber is an extremely important aspect of your diet. Typically, fats, protein, and carbs get all the attention in a diet, but fiber is right up there on the list of important elements in a healthy diet. The amount of fiber in your meal affects the speed at which your body absorbs sugar, meaning it can help reduce the risk of diabetes and high cholesterol.

A simple but accurate tip about fiber is that high fiber foods typically require you to chew them more, taking longer to eat and involving more effort than foods with low fiber contents. If you take your time eating in this manner, your body has more time to recognize that it has received enough food and you are no longer hungry, helping to avoid overeating.

Perhaps the more commonly recognized benefits of eating plenty of fiber are improvements to your gastrointestinal function and health. However, it also helps to prevent some types of cancer, improves your body's glucose tolerance and its response to insulin, and can even lower the risk of hypertension and other heart disease causes.

Summary of Fibers

Soluble Fiber: fruits, oats, barley, legumes

Delays GI transit (benefits digestive disorders)
Delays glucose absorption (benefits diabetics)
Lowers blood cholesterol (benefits heart disease)

Insoluble Fiber: Wheat bran, corn bran, whole grain breads, cereals, cabbage, brussels sprouts
Accelerates GI transit
Promotes healthy bowel movement
Slows starch hydrolysis
Delays glucose absorption

Antioxidants

Your body is in a constant battle against the damage and poison of your environment. In addition to fortifying your body against these dangers by making it physically fit, you can fortify your internal systems by eating the proper foods. Antioxidants are molecules that slow or prevent the damage done to your cells through oxidation. They remove damaging free radicals and are vital to your body's health. Fruits and vegetables are excellent sources of antioxidants and people who eat fruits and vegetables have lower risks of heart disease and some neurological problems as well as several cancers. Green tea and is also a good source of antioxidants.

Brain Food

Your brain cells require twice the amount of energy that your body's other cells need to function, so you need to feed your brain more than facts and figures to keep you and your mental function healthy. As you probably suspect, fruit and vegetables are excellent foods for your brain, but there are other important sources of nutrients that can really benefit your cognitive organ.

Omega-3 fatty acids build and repair your brain and its cells. Fish and nuts have high omega-3 fatty acids amounts, making them great brain food. Yogurt helps your body to create neurotransmitters, which are necessary for proper communication among your brain's neurons. Also, water is essential to your brain's functioning, which is discussed in the chapter on energy tips.

Now that you know what kind of food to eat, you also need to consider what portions and at what intervals you should eat them.

Your Meals

Most people eat 2 fairly large meals a day if that, but if you want to be as healthy, fit, and strong as you can – if you want to really get the most out of this program, you need to eat 5-6 small meals a day, instead. Eating throughout the entire day may seem like an inconvenience, but this change will provide you with incredible and measurable benefits. Eating 5-6 meals a day is surprisingly easy to do and causes changes in the way your body utilizes your food that allow your body to maximize your metabolism and energy potential.

Five to six meals a day instead of 3 allows your body to revert to its natural metabolism, which is much quicker than the rate that large, spaced-out meals has forced your body to create. By raising your metabolism this way, you will quickly begin to lose weight and gain energy with very little effort. Eating two large meals a day prevents your system from being able to efficiently use the calories you eat, sending many of the calories to be stored as fat. Eating more frequently stops this inefficient use of calories, preventing future meals from being stored away as fat, and allows your body to burn off the energy it has stored in the past, melting away your fat.

Similar to the fight or flight reflect mentioned above, your metabolism functions the same now as the metabolism of your long-ago ancestors. Your body and its metabolic processes work to protect you from starvation more than anything else. When you ingest extra calories, your body stores that energy incase you need it someday when you cannot provide yourself with any energy – when you are starving. Your body processes a large meal by using the energy it needs and storing the rest in fat for future use. Since you have food consistently available to you, you are not likely to need this stored energy due to any lack of nutrition.

This is why many fad diets require you to starve yourself. They reason that if you are actually starving, your body will burn away that stored energy and get rid of your fat. However, your body can even protect you in this circumstance, because it adjusts your metabolism according to how much food you are eating. The fewer calories you eat, the fewer calories your body will burn, and the more calories you eat, the more calories your body will burn. This is why starvation-style diets actually cause people to gain weight in the long run.

Weight lost on a fad diet cannot be sustained because these starvation-simulating diets lower your metabolism, promote muscle loss, and eventually shut down your metabolism, directing all the food you eat directly to fat storage.

Your body's primary job is to keep you alive and kicking and your metabolism affects most of your body's vital functions, including your ability to maintain your body temperature, energy levels, glucose levels, hormone levels, and countless other aspects of your well-being. Starvation damages your body's ability to regulate all these things, making starvation-style diets not only unhealthy, but ineffective. Your body will resort to extreme measures to keep you alive and functioning, even if you are just trying to lose weight with your damaging actions.

In order to lose weight and promote muscle growth, you must maintain a diet of lean, high protein, healthy foods six times a day and a rigorous exercise routine. Your body cannot work efficiently without the right quantity and quality of food, and eating 5-6 healthy meals a day can provide your body with exactly what it needs to transform into the body you want. Bodybuilders, models, athletes, and nutrition-aware people use this method of eating in order to achieve the most efficient, healthy, and attractive bodies they can.

If you eat small amounts of healthy food throughout the day, you can experience the benefits of reaching your fitness goals more easily and quickly than if you do not adopt this way of eating. 5-6 meals a day increases your metabolism, raises your energy levels, neutralizes your cravings and hunger pangs, and builds lean muscle mass.

Increasing Your Metabolism with Frequent Meals: The "Thermic Effect" of Food

A person's metabolism is the rate at which he burns the calories he eats. A slow metabolism leads to storage of large amounts of calories as fat, and a fast metabolism burns through the calories of your food as well as potentially any energy stored in your fat. Your metabolic rate is contingent on all sorts of things that you cannot influence, such as your age and sex, but it is also contingent of aspects of your life that you do control. Your muscle mass, which is addressed earlier in this book, changes your metabolism. Also, eating 5-6 meals a day raises your metabolism.

The first way in which eating 5-6 meals a day raises your metabolism is the type of food you eat on this plan. The meals need to be large providers of protein, which not only helps to build your muscles and repair your cells and tissues, but also causes your body to work hard to digest and utilize it. When you eat a lean protein, your body has to chew, digest, break the

152

proteins into individual amino acids, and then rebuild specific chains of amino acids to rebuild the tissues like skin, hair, nails and lean muscle.

For every 100 calories of lean protein ingested we burn 20-25 calories in this process. So this gives us a 20-25% thermic effect from eating lean protein foods. By the way, liquid protein drinks and shakes while nutritious provide little thermic effect compared to real food like fish, chicken breast and lean beef. Carbohydrates will provide a 5-7% thermic effect. Fats on the other hand have only a 3% thermic effect so if you gorge on 2,000 calories from Haagen Daz ice cream, then your body only uses 60 calories to place the fat exactly where you want it the least.

If you ate the same 2,000 calories of lean proteins, fibrous carbs, and starchy carbs, then you could well have used 500 calories in digestion, which will reassure your brain that the body is getting enough calories to avoid starvation while providing a negative calorie balance at the end of the day combined with muscle building exercise, and intervals.

This method of eating stimulates your body's metabolism much more than exercise alone, encouraging your body to burn through stored energy (fat) much more quickly than it would if you were exercising, but still eating your typical 3 meals a day. As mentioned above, eating 5-6 meals a day also stimulates thermogenesis, which raises your metabolism.

Steady Appetite

If you have tried a diet of some sort before, you have probably experienced uncomfortable feelings of hunger and cravings. Most diets require dieters to deny themselves frequent eating or snacks. Eating 6 meals a day, however, prevents feelings of hunger by making you constantly content with the amount of food you are eating.

By eating properly every 2 or 3 hours, you will avoid all these pitfalls of dieting. Regular, small meals keep away cravings and feelings of hunger, helping you to be healthier and happier – there is no need to snack on junk food when you just have and will have again before to long a nice, healthy meal.

If you are more concerned with the fitness than nutrition aspect of this program, then ending food cravings and hunger pains may not be too exciting for you, but keeping away hunger and cravings is actually an invaluable aspect of the 5-6 meals a day program. If you are not already hungry when you are preparing a meal, you are much more likely to recognize your healthy, less readily-available options. Many people grab a snack from the vending machine in the afternoon or while they are cooking dinner, adding unnecessary calories and poor nutritional foods to their day. By eating frequent, healthy meals, however, this determent to your health is easily avoided.

Five to six small meals consisting of a lean protein, complex starchy carb, and fibrous carb are infinitely more beneficial than 3 meals a day, helping you to build muscle, raise your metabolism, and avoid unhealthy, addictive snack foods.

Controlled Blood Sugar and Insulin Equals More Energy

There are many more, internal benefits of eating 5-6 meals a day. Eating 5-6 meals a day, like exercising, helps you body to use energy more efficiently.

Small, frequent meals create a steady, balanced blood sugar level. Your blood sugar level is the amount of glucose, what your cells use for energy, in your blood. Basically, insulin regulates your blood sugar level and how much of it your cells use for energy, so you need insulin to be able to use glucose to have energy. When your blood sugar level drops, you feel an irresistible hunger pang and your energy drops (sound familiar?). Low calories diets and high-carbohydrate snacks cause this effect a lot.

In addition to being inconvenient, these spikes and drops of your energy levels and blood sugar, it is very unhealthy. Eating small, frequent meals, however, helps your body to maintain consistent levels of insulin in our body, properly regulating your blood sugar level and avoiding these drastic peaks and lows altogether. Perhaps you have heard of the importance of insulin and blood sugar regarding diabetes – this method of eating can help to prevent diabetes in addition to helping people who already have it.

Last but not least regarding energy and 5-6 meals a day, you have probably experienced low energy levels after eating a substantial lunch. The reason you feel tired after eating is because your body is working very hard to digest all that food. Your system can handle only so many calories at one time. By eating smaller meals, you are providing your body with much more manageable portions, preventing exhaustion of your body through post-meal strain.

Eating small, frequent meals is the most efficient, effective way to maximize your energy and to provide your body with the quantity and quality of nutrients that you need.

Food for Building Lean Muscle Mass

Changing your eating habits to 5-6 meals a day will be very beneficial to your efforts to build muscle. A regular insulin level – as mentioned above – leads to efficient glucose use. Glucose and amino acids are what support the recovery and growth of your muscles. This means that eating 5-6 meals a day leads to the efficient and effective growth and health of the muscles you are building with your workouts.

Hormones and Their Benefits

You have all sorts of hormones with all sorts of functions. Your hormones influence virtually every aspect of your body's functioning and wellbeing, ranging from how well you sleep and how well you can concentrate to what your hair and skin look like, how hungry you feel, how much energy your body stores as fat, and how much of the stored energy your body burns. Cortisol, insulin, and leptin all deal with your hunger and fat burning and can be beneficially influenced by eating 5-6 meals a day instead of eating 3 meals a day.

Insulin

The hormone insulin dictates to your body the amounts of glucose it should store and produce. As you know, glucose being stored results in fat. Small, frequent meals causes your body to produce less insulin, meaning you will store less of the food you eat as fat.

Cortisol

The hormone cortisol breaks down your muscle mass when your body needs quick energy due to going too long without nutrients. Your body creates cortisol when you have not eaten for a significant amount of time. Furthermore, cortisol is the hormone that moves the extra calories you eat to your fat cells to be stored.

By eating small, frequent meals, you can lessen how much cortisol your body makes. When your body gets used to being consistently provided with the nourishment of 6 meals a day, it does not resort to breaking down your muscles for energy because you are consistently providing it with the energy it needs. Taking a post workout drink of 12-20 grams of whey protein and 16 oz of water will inhibit cortisol following a hard workout.

Leptin

The hormone leptin is created after you eat. Leptin is an appetite suppressant. When you go a significant amount of time without eating, the amount of leptin in your system drops, but when you eat small, frequent meals, your leptin levels are high, avoiding feelings of hunger. Several studies are showing that diet soft drinks, while low in sugar have a tendency to inhibit leptin and therefore will cause you to be hungrier and crave more sugary sweets.

Which Kinds of Food

There are countless benefits to eating 5-6 meals a day, ranging from improved feelings of wellbeing to efficient muscle growth to weight loss. This way of eating is the healthiest, most efficient way to provide your body with the nutrients and energy it needs.

Of course, frequent feedings does not mean you will be eating twice as much food as you do now or that you can eat unhealthy meals. Eating this way, you will consume basically the same amount of food as you did before or slightly more, and these meals will consist of the most beneficial food for your fitness.

In order to promote lean muscle mass, high energy, and general health, these meals should consist of lean meats high in protein, complex and fibrous carbohydrates, vegetables, fruits, and healthy amounts of whole grains. You need to include healthy fats, but avoid carbohydrates that are high on the glycemic index.

Protein shakes are a great way to eat some of your meals that you feel you are too busy to take the time for. Remember that while a liquid meal replacement is better than skipping a meal, it doesn't provide the thermic calorie burning effect of eating real food.

Other good foods for this program include chicken breasts, turkey, tuna, salmon, brown rice, nuts (in small amounts), and seeds. I have included lists of foods that are perfect for your 6 meals a day diet as well as a food log for you.

Nutritional Information

Supportive Eating Examples

Lean Proteins	Starchy Carbohydrates	Fibrous Carbohydrates
Eggs	Potato	Broccoli
Shellfish	Cream of rice cereal	Onions
Sea Bass	Corn	Cauliflower
Chicken breast	Brown rice	Asparagus
Sushi/Sashimi	Sweet potato	Carrots
Turkey breast	Peas	Spinach
Halibut	Basmati rice	Green peppers
Tuna	Oatmeal	String beans
Tilapia	Couscous	Bell peppers
Shrimp	Corn tortillas	Cucumbers
Grouper	Whole grain breads	Mushrooms
Lobster	Whole grain pastas	Artichokes
Mahi Mahi	Cream of wheat	Cabbage
Cod	cereal	Brussels sprouts
Lean Beef	Black beans	Kale
Salmon	Wheatina	Turnips
Fat-free dairy	Pinto beans	Scallions
products		Arugula
Swordfish		Romaine lettuce
Veal		Zucchini
		Most vegetables
Fruits (are high glycemic so be sure to eat only with a lean protein.)	apples blueberries strawberries melons bananas	

160

When filling out your nutrition log, look for an item from each category for your main meals and a protein and fibrous carb for your snacks. I substitute my fruits at breakfast and snack time. After the first week or two, it will not be necessary to weigh or measure every food item since you should be able to eyeball the portions.

Finding Food Values and Reliable Information

There is not enough space in this book to list all the nutrients in foods, but you can very easy use online sources to get this for yourself when choosing items for your meals. You will not have to do this after the first few weeks due to familiarity with the meals.

The following are a few websites I recommend for nutritional and reliable fat loss information:

www.drlenkravitz.com -- Dr. Kravitz is the head of the exercise physiology department at the University of New Mexico. At his site you will find extremely helpful information about proven methods to help you. He is also writes in a style that is very easy to understand.

www.alwincosgrove.com -- If you want to know everything there is to know about fat loss in no B.S. presentation then be prepared for a roller coaster ride of laughing and learning.

www.nutribase.com -- Go there and download the free USDA database of nutrients for most foods. It is very complete and their only free download. They also have a comprehensive individual diet program for 49.95.

www.nutritiontrainer.com -- This is the best tool for analyzing and preparing nutritionally sound menus for you and your family. It is very user friendly and you will be amazed at how simple it is to add foods that will complete a meal and subtract those that will interfere with your progress.

www.tomincledon.com -- Tom Incledon is one of the few nutritional geniuses in the world today and has a section where you can find out if a supplement you might consider taking is any good or a waste of money.

www.philkaplan.com -- Phil's site is a wealth of fitness and supplement information. It is easy to navigate and entertaining to read. Most of those who train with Coach Terry will say that they have heard me preach the same fitness truth.

www.nal.usda.gov/fnic/foodcomp/search -- This is the USDA national nutrient database. When you type in a food it lists 3 oz. or 100 gram portions of the specific food along with calories, fats, carbs, vitamins, and minerals.

www.powereating.com -- Susan Kliener is one of the world's top experts on nutrition. This is her website.

I also recommend the *Salter Nutri-Scale*. This scale gives the calories, protein, fat, and carbs for many foods, based on the actual weight of the food on the scale. I found mine at Bed Bath and Beyond and thought it was worth showing all of my clients.

How to Use the Food Log

Make keeping a log easy on yourself. If you find that you are going to too much trouble to track calories, just list your foods that you eat for each meal. If you find that you are not losing fat, then adjust your portion sizes.

Fill in all of the fields. If you did not have a lean protein, starchy carb, or fibrous carb during a meal or snack, then write none. By keeping track, you will be able to more clearly see what you may be missing on a regular basis. Also, list your supplements at the bottom of the pages in the daily total area.

Drink water all day. A few small sips every 15-20 minutes will benefit you by keeping you hydrated, assisting in fat loss and lubricating your complexion and joints.

On the following pages are sample and blank Food Logs. If you want more food and exercise log pages, you have my permission to copy them and use them in good health.

Supportive Nutrition Sample   Date: _____

Food, Drink and Supplements Consumed	Total calories	Protein grams 4	Carbs grams 4	Fat grams 9
Meal 1:				
1/3 cup non-fat yogurt	495	5	27	2.5
½ cup soymilk, 2 tbsp nuts (LP)		1.1	23	0.3
½ cup oatmeal (SC)		1.8	0.8	4.6
½ cup blueberries* (FC)		7	8.3	4
12 oz coffee, 1 tbsp cream (H₂0)		Trace	17.3	0
Meal 2:				
3 tbsp almond butter (P,F)	303	7.2	10	28.2
2 slices whole wheat bread (SC)	130	5	23.6	2
1 tbsp blackberry jam (S)	6	0	13.7	0
Water				
Meal 3:				
4 oz white meat turkey (LP)	240	32	0	11
2 slices whole wheat bread (SC)	130	5	23.6	2
2 slices of tomato (FC)	6	0.1	1.2	0
½ cup of spinach (FC)	20	2.65	3.37	0
Meal 4:				
½ oz (11) almonds (P,F)	80	3	2.7	7
1 apple	71	0.3	19	0
Meal 5:				
4 oz baked salmon (LP)	240	24	0	14
1 cup steamed broccoli (FC)	54	2.8	11	0.6
½ baked sweet potato (6 oz)	60	1.2	12.5	0
12 oz Water				
Meal 6:				
Total Grams:		95.5	193.7	76.2
Total Calories:	1815	382	774.8	

LP: Lean Protein / **SC:** Starchy Carbs / **FC:** Fibrous Carbs / **P,F:** Protein, Fat / **S:** Sugar

Supportive Nutrition   Date: _____

Food, Drink and Supplements Consumed	Total calories	Protein grams 4	Carbs grams 4	Fat grams 9
BREAKFAST Lean protein: Starchy carb: Fibrous carb: Water:				
SNACK Lean protein: Starchy carb: Fibrous carb: Water:				
LUNCH Lean protein: Starchy carb: Fibrous carb: Water:				

(Continued on next page)

SNACK Lean protein: Starchy carb: Fibrous carb: Water:				
DINNER Lean protein: Starchy carb: Fibrous carb: Water:				
SNACK Lean protein: Starchy carb: Fibrous carb: Water:				
Daily Totals				
What I did well:				
What I would like to improve:				

Sticking With It

One of the comments I hear regularly is this: "I've been on the best programs and haven't seen any results after working so hard. What is wrong?

The best way to answer this is that either the program actually wasn't one of the best like we discussed earlier. (It doesn't work) Another is that you may have adapted. Finally either by choice or unconsciously you may not be following the program, or given it enough time to work.

Quite simply if you are not losing at a rate that you are comfortable with you need to re-evaluate your program, and stick with it. You do need to give any changes you make time to work however. You can't change something and expect your body to adjust overnight - give everything time to work.

Recommended Reading

Transform and *The Best You've Ever Been* by Phil Kaplan
Phil Kaplan's book is reader friendly and provides plenty of effective tips, and a 17 week program to change your body.

Eating for Life by Bill Phillips
Bill Phillips provides over 20 supportive breakfasts, lunches and dinners with recipes and pictures of all you need to build a fantastic meal plan that will stoke your metabolism and delight your appetite.

Power Eating by Susan Kliener, Rd. PhD
Susan Kliener will explain the most complex concepts regarding weight management in a way that anyone can understand and apply. She also gives the truth about many supplements that are useful or not for your program.

The Essence of Program Design by Juan Carlos Santana (for coaches, personal trainers, and athletes)

Afterburn by Alwyn Cosgrove
Alwyn is the mad genius of the fitness world and is one of the few who can make you laugh while learning how to apply the latest fitness and fat loss knowledge to your successful efforts.

Summary and a Few (more) Words

Much of what we've learned can be condensed into a few paragraphs so that you can be empowered to create any fitness or body related result that you desire for the rest of your life.
Remember to combine strength training, cardio based intervals, cardio for health, and supportive nutrition.
Eat a lean protein, fibrous carbohydrate, and small starchy carbohydrate at every meal.
Avoid sugar, since it is your worst enemy if you wish to lose fat.
Everything else is details and instructions.

Keep in mind that by following the guidelines presented in this book, you will own the power to control your metabolism, weight management, bone density, and reduced risk of lifestyle related diseases associated with aging.

I am always delighted to hear from readers interested in fitness and health. Feel free to send questions to terry@coachterrysfitness.com

Exercise safely at all times and have fun with it.

Glossary

Antioxidant Vitamins and nutrients that repair cell damage caused by oxidation. Vitamins C, E, and A, which is a derivative of beta carotene, are examples of antioxidants.

Basal Metabolic Rate (BMR) is the amount of energy you burn while you are physically at rest. This accounts for approximately 70 percent of the energy you burn in a day and is composed of the energy burned by your body's organs and systems.

Blood Sugar Level is the amount of sugar, or glucose, in your blood.

Bodybuilding is the process of maximizing muscle hypertrophy through the combination of weight training, sufficient caloric intake, and rest, often utilizing extraneous hormones. Someone who engages in this activity is referred to as a bodybuilder. The muscles are revealed through a combination of fat loss, oils, and tanning (or tanning lotions), which combine with lighting to make the definition of the muscle group more distinct.

Calorie A measurement for the energy provided for your body by the food you eat. Your body burns your food's calories to provide it with the energy it needs. The energy you feed your body that it does not need gests stored as fat.

Carbohydrates All plant foods and some dairy products contain carbohydrates, also known as carbs. Carbs are composed of sugar molecules that, if eaten properly, give your body energy and nourishment. Your body converts your food's carbs into glucose, which energizes your cells. The extra carbs you eat are made into glycogen, which is stored as fat.

Cardiovascular Exercise Also known as cardio, cardiovascular exercise is intense exercise that requires you to breathe hard. This aerobic exercise strengthens your circulatory and respiratory health as well as your heart and lungs.

Cholesterol is a type of fat in your body's cells. Cholesterol is necessary for your body to carry out many important processes, including the creation of hormones – including testosterone and adrenaline – cell membrane structure construction, use of vitamin D, and efficient metabolism function. Your body creates cholesterol on its own, so you do not need to include cholesterol in your diet to be able to perform these functions.

Complex Carbohydrate are the "good" carbohydrates made of sugar and found in the starches and fibers of legumes, whole grains, and starchy vegetables. Complex carbs have healthy vitamins, minerals, and fiber.

Exercise Different exercises involve moving joints in specific patterns to challenge muscles in different ways to gain strength and endurance.

Fiber slows the rates of your body's sugar absorption when you eat. Slowing this rate can help to reduce your risk of diabetes. A diet with plenty of fiber can also lower cholesterol and prevent constipation.

Form Each exercise has a specific form, or topography of movement designed to maximize safety and muscle strength gains.

Glucose is the energy-providing sugar in blood. Although glucose is vital to your energy levels, excess glucose is stored as fat.

Glycemic Index (GI) This index rates how quickly foods' carbohydrates are converted into glucose. A high rating on the glycemic index means a food converts the carbohydrates quickly, causing the sugar to enter your blood more quickly, and, consequently, quickly raising your blood sugar level.

High Density Lipoprotein Cholesterol (HDL) is also known as "good" cholesterol. HDL helps your body to remove "bad" cholesterol (LDL) from your bloodstream.

Insulin The hormone that tells your body's system how much glucose to make and store.

Metabolism The rate that you burn calories.

Monounsaturated Fats Lower the amounts of bad cholesterol in your system and increase your amounts of good cholesterol. Monounsaturated fats can be found in avocado, nuts, and canola and olive oil.

Muscle Mass You build the amount of muscle in your body by exercising, which increases your muscle mass. Muscle mass burns energy at all times, including when you are physical inactive. This means that muscle mass burns much, much more calories than fat does, so the more muscle mass you have, the more calories you will burn in a day.

Muscle Tone Residual muscle tension or tonus is the continuous and passive partial contraction of the muscles. Tone helps maintain posture and declines during REM sleep. Note that muscular tone is not defined as muscular shaping or the aspect of general human physical appearance. Unconscious nerve impulses maintain the muscles in a partially contracted state. If a sudden pull or stretch occurs, the body responds by automatically increasing the muscle's tension. This reflex helps guard against danger as well as helps maintain balance.

Polyunsaturated Fats Found in seafood, soy, corn, and sunflower oils. This "good" fat lowers bad cholesterol.

Protein is a vital element of your body's health. Your diet must include protein in order to be able to repair and build your cells, tissue, and muscles.

Rep is short for repetition. A rep is a single cycle of lifting and lowering a certain weight in a controlled manner, moving through the form of the exercise.

Saturated Fats This "bad" fat raises your bad cholesterol. Most animal products and some plant products include saturated fat, including meant, butter, coconut oil, and eggs.

Set A set consists of several repetitions performed one after another with no break between them and with the number of reps per set and sets per exercise depending on the goal of the individual.

Simple Carbohydrates are also known as simple sugars. These carbohydrates are made of sugar and can be found in fruit, dairy products, and candy. They are often called "bad" carbohydrates because of their low nutritional value and high calorie content.

Tempo is the speed with which an exercise is performed. The tempo of a movement has implications for the weight that can be moved and the effects on the muscle.

Thermogenesis Your body's process for creating internal heat.

Trans Fat An unnatural fat that was created in a lab to lengthen foods' shelf lives and to make them more capable of withstanding the production process. Trans fat is found mostly in packaged foods, snacks, junk food, margarines, and commercially fried food.

Weight Training is a common type of strength training for developing the strength and size of skeletal muscles. Weight training uses the force of gravity in the form of weighted bars, dumbbells, or weight stacks to oppose the force generated by muscle through concentric or eccentric contraction. Weight training uses a variety of specialized equipment to target specific muscle groups and types of movement.

Index

Printed in the United States
128646LV00003B/172-249/P

9 780981 890005